PRAISE FOR
THE WEB-SAVVY PATIENT

"*Andrew Schorr has used the positive aspects of the Web – first to connect people with his* Patient Power *programs and now with this book – to filter the near endless collective human knowledge into serviceable portions. He is helping health care by bringing informed patients and their health care providers closer together.*"

Jens R. Chapman, M.D.

Acting Chair, Department of Orthopaedic Surgery and Sports Medicine
University of Washington

"*Andrew Schorr is a gifted communicator who is able to translate medical information into language everyone can understand. In this book, he provides a gateway for patients to improve and optimize their care with a Web-savvy approach, which will likely lead them to better outcomes.*"

James R. Berenson, M.D.

Chief Executive Officer, President and Medical and Scientific Director
Institute for Myeloma and Bone Cancer Research

"The Web-Savvy Patient *draws from Andrew Schorr's own experiences as a patient with a serious illness, a reporter and a medical communicator. He writes from the heart with insight and hard-earned knowledge.*"

Tom Linden, M.D.
Director, Medical and Science Journalism Program
University of North Carolina at Chapel Hill

"*It is rare to find personal patient experience, Web-based medical guidance and easy-to-follow health content in a single source. Schorr beautifully demonstrates how people looking to take charge of their health care can use the Internet as a valuable resource for understanding, coping and obtaining guidance.*"

Nehal N. Mehta, M.D., M.S., FACP, FAHA
Director of Inflammatory Risk, Preventive Cardiology
University of Pennsylvania School of Medicine

"Trying to navigate medical information on the Web can be overwhelming and take time away from one's personal recovery process. The Web-Savvy Patient helps patients focus on obtaining the most useful resources and advocating for their own best health. This accelerates the healing process, which is the most important benefit of all."

Pat Elliott

E-patient advocate and cancer survivor

"Nowadays the Internet is the first stop for anyone handed a serious diagnosis. This treasure trove of well-informed common sense can help patients, families and friends make the most of the Internet, as well as cope with the emotional turmoil of dealing with life-and-death decisions."

Peter Frishauf

Founder, Medscape

THE

WEB-SAVVY
PATIENT

An Insider's Guide to
Navigating the Internet
When Facing Medical Crisis

Andrew Schorr

with
Mary Adam Thomas

ISBN: 1456324993
ISBN-13: 9781456324995
LCCN: 2010916787

www.WebSavvyPatient.com

TABLE OF CONTENTS

FOREWORD

By Michael J. Keating, M.B., B.S.

I work as a physician at one of the major cancer centers in the world. Patients who come to our center are either fortunate enough to live in the surrounding area of Houston or have found their way to us through a massive maze of information. They have searched for the physicians and centers that have true expertise in their particular disease. Often times, the search is not made by the patients (who tend to be older) but by their children and even grandchildren who search the Internet to find the best treatment for their father, mother, grandfather, grandmother, aunt, uncle or child.

The tech-savvy patient often arrives in the doctor's office with a binder of various bits of information from the Internet. Many have quotes from chat pages or Internet sites. The information quality ranges from outstanding to destructive.

It is rare to find a collection of information that is relevant. I think that Andrew Schorr's personal journey has led him to a vocation that truly empowers patients and gives them the greatest opportunity to find centers of excellence within their reach. It is easy to say, "When I get the diagnosis of a serious illness – cancer, heart disease, neurologic disease, etc. – I will check it out on the Internet." When the diagnosis is made, however, the patient's mind in many ways shuts down. They are often terrified of the prospect of what has been portrayed to them with their diagnosis and terrified of making a wrong decision.

Preventive medicine has moved to the forefront as a topic of conversation. I agree that it is time for us to consider preventive information. *The Web-Savvy Patient* is a wonderful book to read after the diagnosis is made, but it also will benefit those who have not yet experienced a significant diagnosis. This book will help in forward planning for people in the middle or later phases of their life to get accurate, focused, relevant and current information before a diagnosis of a serious illness is made.

It is rare to find an author who is both altruistic and knowledgeable. Andrew is one of them. As his physician, I have been constantly amazed at his passion to empower patients in their decision making. Health care is really the interaction between the patient and the doctor with supporting professionals and institutions. Andrew's book shows you the right way to conduct this interaction for the greater benefit of both the patient and the physician and, eventually, our entire health care program.

Michael J. Keating, M.B., B.S.

Professor of Medicine and Internist

Department of Leukemia, Division of Cancer Medicine

The University of Texas MD Anderson Cancer Center

A WORD OF CAUTION

This book is not intended to offer clinical advice or guidance. It is meant to provide support for those patients and caregivers who want to use the Internet in their quest for information and empowerment. When facing a serious illness or health condition, seek professional medical attention immediately.

How to Read This Book

The Web-Savvy Patient contains words of patient wisdom delivered in multiple forms. In each section of the book you will find:

- Practical guidance through objective information.
- Personal, subjective points of view from real patients.
- True stories of empowered patients.

Anyone facing a life-changing diagnosis will recognize elements of his or her own story on some of the pages of this book.

Here's how to find what you need:

INTRODUCTION

An overview of Andrew Schorr's leukemia diagnosis, treatment, remission and survivorship that will help you get oriented and relate to the perspective of the lead author. This section also examines how Andrew's role as a cancer patient altered the course of his professional life as a medical journalist/educator, and how both were affected by the emergence of the Internet. A serious diagnosis changes you – Andrew's story is one example – but may give you a clue to the changes that could be coming.

CHAPTERS ONE THROUGH TEN

Subject-specific guides from an insider's viewpoint. Packed with how-to information, practical tips and examples of real patients whose self-advocacy played a part in their medical journeys and, in most cases, led them to better care. Each of these chapters focuses on one aspect of how the Internet can be a life-saving tool, beginning with the segment of Andrew's story that pertains to the subject of that chapter.

The Web offers a world of medical information to help you be what Andrew likes to call a "powerful patient." This book will not only guide you in your online activities but also help you with what you may do offline to organize and apply the information in your interactions with your doctor, other patients, family and friends. The Internet is only one part of your arsenal as a powerful patient and should be integrated with other tools. However, your online research and "Web-savvy" approach can only help put you in a stronger position to receive better care and the hope for better health.

THE CONVERSATION CONTINUES ONLINE

Your journey as a patient is as dynamic as the Internet. This book will provide framework and guidance for your quest for information but was written at a single point in time. Continue your discoveries as a powerful patient by joining the book's online community at **www.WebSavvyPatient.com**, where you will find updates, videos and more. The website serves as a gathering place for the patients and family members for whom this book is just the beginning.

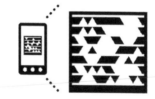

Get the free mobile app at http://gettag.mobi then point your Web-enabled device at this code to connect to www.WebSavvyPatient.com.

{ INTRODUCTION }

ANDREW'S STORY

From Reporter to Patient to Survivor to Advocate

I am a man who was at the wrong place at the right time. I received a diagnosis that changed my life. Now my hope is that what I have learned and the people I have met can change yours.

You are most likely reading this because you or someone you care about is facing a medical crisis. We are not talking about tennis elbow or poison ivy. We are talking about serious medical conditions – the kind where the diagnosis shakes you emotionally and you wonder whether life is over, or over as you've known it or hoped it would be.

This book can be your best friend as you turn, maybe in the middle of the night, to where most people now go when facing a life-changing diagnosis. They no longer rely just on the doctor or hospital, but also on the Internet. It may be patients searching for themselves to gain understanding and calm their fears, or it could be a spouse or an adult child of someone facing illness.

Let me tell you how it began for me and how my journey – and the timing of it – has put me in a unique position to write this book with the hope of helping you.

One early April morning in 1996, I was just finishing my usual three-mile run near my home on Mercer Island, Washington, outside of Seattle. It was clear, sunny and cool. I was celebrating the endorphin rush a runner can get and was slowing down as I ran down the hill to my house. Kasha, my black lab and running companion, was panting. I was ready for the day.

I touched my nose, which I thought was running. There was blood on my hand. One part of me was thinking it was no big deal. A nose bleed could happen on a crisp morning. But another voice said to me, "Is this the way it starts? Is this the beginning of the end?"

I told no one. Then it happened again a day or so later. I called my HMO clinic and was given an appointment the same day with my very dry, very British internist, Dr. Peter Littlewood. He was a no-baloney veteran doctor. And being at an HMO, he was happy to tell people that 99 times out of 100 their fears were unwarranted.

"It's probably nothing," he said as he used a scope to peer into my nose. He didn't see anything to cauterize, no blood vessels too close to the surface. So he ordered a blood test. He was wondering if my platelets (the cells that promote clotting) were low.

"I'll only call you if it's serious," he said as I left for the lab. He smiled as if to project some certainty that this healthy, middle-aged runner wouldn't be hearing from him anytime soon. I could only hope.

Later that day, I was sitting at my desk at my downtown Seattle health communications company where we made videos for patients and doctors. We'd also developed innovative talk shows over the phone for patients with chronic conditions like multiple sclerosis and asthma.

The phone rang. The receptionist said Dr. Littlewood was on the line. My heart immediately sped up. "How do you feel?" he asked. I told him I felt fine. "You haven't had the flu or a cold?" he pressed on. I told him no. I felt great. I'll never forget Dr. Littlewood responding, "That's not what I wanted to hear."

I asked him what this was all about. He explained my white blood count was elevated like I was fighting an infection or had recently. My platelets were fine. He wanted to retest. "When?" I asked. "Right away," came the clipped response. My head was spinning as I drove back to the clinic.

I became a journalist many years before. I was a television news reporter in Charlotte and Los Angeles, with a stop as a national reality television producer in San Francisco.

I had covered many medical subjects, and I had certainly heard medical tests could be wrong. I was eager to rush back to the clinic to get more accurate numbers. I was home that night and had not said a word to Esther, my wife and partner in Schorr Communications, when Dr. Littlewood called again. The blood test results were the same. "It could be a leukemia," he said. I was reeling. Spring was approaching, but I suddenly saw myself withering away.

I had no clear understanding of leukemia as a blood cancer, nor any knowledge that there were different types. I had heard of the Leukemia Society, probably given money for research when a neighbor came by. But I never, ever thought I would become a leukemia patient at 45 and be facing death from such a diagnosis.

Esther is my best friend as well as my spouse. She can be an emotionally charged person. I am much more even-keeled – my typical m.o. from being in some dicey situations as a news reporter and having to remain calm. I had to tell her that night about what my doctor had said and I did.

Dr. Littlewood told me I was being referred to an oncologist. Within a day or so, Esther and I were there as that doctor, Dr. Eric Feldman, confirmed my diagnosis of chronic lymphocytic leukemia or CLL. He said it was the "good kind" of leukemia to have since it typically progresses slowly. But the bad news was it was incurable and would shorten my life, bringing death from an infection that my damaged immune system would eventually be unable to fight off.

Perhaps as with your experience, there were plenty of tears, disbelief and sadness. I did not know what I would say to my two children. Our eldest, Ari, was 6. Ruthie was just 2.

Esther and I took a long walk in the woods that afternoon. I remember feeling I was at peace if this was the end. I had lived fully, although not long enough. My wife, I am happy to say, was not ready to let me go.

We had a sense that information could help us gain some control, bolster us with a better understanding of my situation than what the doctor provided as he gave us the "bad news." Esther remembered that our friend David Nudelman thrived on searching on the Internet and participating in "news groups." I had no understanding of what they were or how to find them, let alone how to join one if somewhere there were people like me, diagnosed with a disease I had never heard of before.

Esther called David and he was at our home computer within an hour or so. After just a few keystrokes, David had found a "listserv," an online community of people with blood cancers around the world sending messages to and from each other through a central computer system. Here were my guides – people who had gone before me and, we came to realize, were ready to help someone new.

This patient-to-patient connection in the early days of the Internet not only changed the course of my treatment, it amped up the purpose for my life. Strange, but I was already in health communications – a niche that made sense to me coming out of my broader journalism experience. (I began as a television news reporter in Charlotte, N.C. in 1972.) Now I was a patient too, just like the people I served in health communications. I was living the same pain now, and

I had a duty, if I survived, to use my skill to help make things better for others.

That has come to pass. This book – created with my long-time friend and colleague, writer Mary Adam Thomas – is part of that purpose. I had already hatched the ideas for talk shows for patients in 1996 and was delivering them via conference call technology. I had just started to see if we could also "stream" the audio on a website. I quickly lined up financial support to do that for my new community of people with CLL. World famous experts and patients quickly signed on to speak or to listen.

That connection further affected my individual care. I learned about clinical trials. I learned that not all doctors were on the leading edge or especially attentive to my fairly uncommon condition. My Internet broadcast programs in CLL helped me realize I had to use what I was learning and take action. I had to feel empowered. That meant going back to Dr. Feldman and telling him I wanted to travel to another city to consult with a CLL specialist. There was none at the time in Seattle, my home city. Dr. Feldman didn't balk at the idea, but said that the HMO would not pay for that second opinion.

This was my life on the line! How could I not invest in my health by going the extra mile? So Esther and I flew to Houston and the University of Texas M. D. Anderson Cancer Center, a huge facility devoted to only cancer that was bigger than most hospitals that treat many illnesses.

We found ourselves in a city we had never visited before and where we knew no one, scheduled to see a doctor we had never heard of before – all because of that community back on the Internet. They told us where to go, whom to see, where to stay. And before long, some Houston locals from the Internet even joined us for lunch and dinner. We discovered we were not alone. We had knowing guides locally and others waiting for word online.

Our listserv mentors had recommended Dr. Michael Keating, a world renowned CLL specialist. He turned out to be a genial man with a broad smile and ready bear hugs. I underwent extensive testing in the morning of my visit, and Esther and I saw Dr. Keating in the mid-afternoon. He greeted us with a big smile and quickly assured us I wasn't dying any time soon. Maybe the CLL would never become aggressive. That happens in a minority of cases. Or, if it did advance, he might have better treatments when it did. But the bottom line was: no treatment now.

I was both shocked and happy to hear that. It was the exact opposite of what Dr. Feldman had recommended as a plan. He had even predicted Dr. Keating would agree with that course of treatment. "Hell no!" Dr. Keating said in person. "Maybe I would have recommended that a year or two ago, but we are way past that now."

So the best plan, according to Dr. Keating, was to "watch and wait." "Watch and worry" is what my pals on the Internet called it.

More was revealed in that exam room that changed our life. Esther explained we had hoped to have a third child but were reconsidering because of my diagnosis. Dr. Keating gave Esther one of his trademark big bear hugs.

"Go have your baby," he said. "Andrew will be with us a long, long time."

We did have a baby the next year. And four years later, I entered Dr. Keating's clinical trial. Now we have Eitan, a testosterone-filled, football-playing kid. And I take no medicine; the leukemia cells are no longer detectable. Once again I feel great.

What we found on the Internet gave Eitan life and gave a second one to his dad.

I continued to work in online health communications while undergoing treatment over six months from 2000 to 2001 with standard chemotherapy and Dr. Keating's experimental medicine. I worked with doctors, hospitals and drug companies producing content related to a wide array of health conditions. Schorr Communications became HealthTalk.com. In the waning days of the Internet boom, millions of dollars in venture capital came in (to give greater life to what we started, even if I became sicker). Esther and I were no longer in control, the money people were, but I got to participate in online health communications and become savvy about the forces at work there. My push was to put patients first and give them a loud voice in their care.

Fifty people eventually worked at HealthTalk, and then the company was sold to another organization tied to pharmaceutical marketing, then it was sold again to become part of the major consumer health website, EverydayHealth.com. Along the way, I met or talked to hundreds of people involved in online offerings to consumers like you. Some had patients' best interests at heart. Some did not. I was well aware that many doctors warn patients that they have to be careful of health information on the Web.

That is true. But patient-to-patient connections online have helped me and they can help you too. So can online connections with medical experts and medical information. You just need a helping hand from a savvy guide to help you navigate the Web. The next pages will give you just that, with specific recommendations from me and from people I respect.

This book has emerged over the past four years. It was in February 2005 that I detached myself from HealthTalk and created "Patient Power." I wanted to host a radio talk show and maybe host television segments too, covering medical topics from the patient's perspective. I hoped these shows would be featured by Seattle media and maybe on a network like CNN.

I was dreaming, because no news manager took the bait. However, a major talk radio station in Seattle offered an alternative. If I would buy an hour or two of weekly radio time, they'd be happy to put me on the air. I chafed at the idea of paying them to bring a much-needed patient perspective that was already taking hold on the Internet but was nowhere to be found on radio or TV – and still isn't.

But I bit the bullet. I had to commit a sizable amount of money for one hour of Sunday morning radio air time for over one year and I had to say yes within a few days. Was I willing to risk a chunk of my retirement savings for this mission? I hoped I could get sponsors to offset the cost, but I decided I could not turn away from this unusual "opportunity."

The good news is that my friends at the University of Washington quickly agreed to sponsor the program. (I had partnered with them previously at HealthTalk.) Then another major hospital signed on, and another. The University of Washington remains Patient Power's biggest sponsor today as we have expanded to worldwide live and on-demand Internet talk shows on PatientPower.info. Leaders at the University of Washington feel that patient empowerment, led by a patient, is consistent with their mission. Several other elite medical centers have joined in, including M. D. Anderson. I am very grateful.

I have had the rare opportunity to interview some of America's most inspiring patients and most knowledgeable medical experts. These individuals participated because they wanted accurate, empowering information online for people like you. Their hope, and mine, is that they can become a loud voice to cut through the clutter of online sites that try to sell you something, cheat you or send you on a wild goose chase.

I have hosted hundreds of webcasts, town meetings and interviews. Plus, I have been writing about my perspective on health issues and events, often with the topic triggered by an event in my life, a chance meeting or a topic in the news. This first started as a personal journal while beginning treatment for my leukemia in 2000 and continued as blogging as of 2005. I invite you to browse through the blog archives at PatientPower.info to see if you can find something that pertains to your situation.

For this book, we've woven together insightful information with the stories of scores of path-finding patients and caregivers. I hope you'll find this a fine mix of facts and "heart," because you are not just on a clinical journey, you are on an emotional one too. I hope *The Web-Savvy Patient* will become your guide to online health, enabling you to join the growing ranks of powerful patients.

Yes, I was at the wrong place at the right time – leukemia at the dawn of online health. Surviving cancer has indeed changed my life. By sharing my Internet skills with a wider audience through the creation of this book, I hope to make a difference. Maybe that's why I survived.

So begin the journey in these pages toward understanding online medical information and its great potential to assist you in this difficult time. No one knows what the health result will be for you. But I congratulate you for trying to get accurate information, whether you are a patient, a caregiver or a friend. This approach led me to better health, and I pray it will do the same for you.

Andrew Schorr
Mercer Island, Washington
January 2011

{ One }

Identifying the Problem

Find Out What's Going On

In my experience

The day I was diagnosed with leukemia, I felt completely overwhelmed and under-informed. I was aware that leukemia was bad — really bad — but I didn't even fully understand that it was a type of cancer. All I knew was that I associated it with illness and death. So if I had it, I assumed I would surely die. My mind raced in those first few hours following my diagnosis. I did what most people do in similar situations: jump to dangerous and frightening conclusions while armed with very little information.

What I did not understand in that earliest phase of my life as a leukemia patient was how to distinguish my own situation from those of all other individuals falling under the leukemia category. I hadn't yet learned the important distinctions between chronic and acute forms of the disease or the many variations of the condition that make such a significant difference when it comes to treatment and prognosis.

I began my online research at a time when the Internet was in its infancy and my comprehension of my condition was minimal. Still, I embarked on the journey determined to find answers. I quickly discovered that my first challenge was figuring out which questions to ask.

FIRST THINGS FIRST

You have just received diagnostic news from a physician. You or a loved one has been labeled with something that sounds like a death sentence. What now?

For most of us, receiving a serious diagnosis is a chaotic, confusing and scary experience. Whether you are the patient or the caregiver, you can't help but feel worried if the condition is one with which you have little or no familiarity.

Our instincts tell us to gather as much data as possible as quickly as possible in order to become

Insider's Tip:

Approach your online research as you would any important data-gathering project. Be thorough and discriminating.

better informed. These days, that means heading straight to the Internet. But when it comes to medical crises, the Web can be just as harmful as helpful because it can lead to incorrect and/or irrelevant information. In your early days as an empowered patient, you must begin your quest for answers using the proper road map.

Do not let fear and panic drive your research. Try to remember that knowledge is power. The greater your sense of calm, the greater your ability to gather and digest the information that will assist you. The goal is to arm yourself with wisdom that will allow you to be a strong, active participant in your own care.

The good and bad news about the Internet is that it offers both up-to-the-minute and archived content, which can be confusing for patients researching medical conditions. The latest and greatest – and most hopeful – treatment options for certain conditions are lumped with outdated statistics that convey what might be a much grimmer outcome.

In my case, an acquaintance told me that she had read about leukemia being "an always fatal condition." But leukemia as a disease category includes numerous sub-categories, each of which comes with its own set of challenges, treatments and prognoses.

Insider's Tip:

Remember that there are millions of pages on the Internet that are out of date and never deleted.

One must always wade through facts and figures, paying attention only to data that is applicable and up-to-date. Researching a medical condition involves a lot of detective work. You may certainly start with Wikipedia or other general information sites, but it is imperative that you use them only as starting points. You might begin at this top tier of the Internet, but go into it knowing that you'll need to drill farther down into the lower levels of the Web until you reach sites that are clinically relevant to your particular case.

CONDITION VS. EMERGENCY

This book is devoted to the patient-side research and management of chronic medical conditions, rather than acute medical emergencies. In the thick of most "911 situations," the Internet plays less of a role, if any at all. So be sure not to turn to the computer when you should be calling for immediate medical assistance if an emergency arises. If an emergency leads to a diagnosis, you can use the Web in all the ways described in these chapters.

A LESSON IN LISTENING TO YOUR GUT

Sometimes patient empowerment is a matter of paying attention to your instincts. That was true for Beth Mays of Houston, the first of the individuals we'll meet in these pages whose true story demonstrates the potentially life-saving importance of hunting for definitive information. She began as a trusting mom with a sick kid. When she wasn't getting answers and her son wasn't getting better, she was transformed into a feisty patient advocate and a national leader for other families.

Mother's intuition told Beth that her infant son, Charlie, was dealing with something more serious than what doctors repeatedly told her was nothing to worry about. Charlie had always been a fussy baby who spit up more than Beth's three older children had. He screamed as if in agony, sometimes for hours on end. His vomiting episodes slowly escalated to the point where he would become violently ill eight to ten times a day. Still, his pediatrician insisted it was "just a little bug" and accused Beth of being an anxious mother. He agreed to run some tests but they provided no answers, so Beth and Charlie were sent on their way.

After a difficult three-month stretch with no relief, Beth took Charlie to the emergency room, where she thought she could get her son the attention he needed. The first doctor to examine Charlie repeated the "it's just a bug" line, but another doctor took notice. The next day, Charlie, then 16 months old, was admitted. Three days later, a gastroen-terologist found that Charlie's esophagus was 50 percent swollen and inflamed, his stomach and small intestines had open sores and his digestive system had shut down.

Charlie began to receive total parenteral nutrition (TPN), which involved putting a feeding tube directly into his body. Multiple IV lines were hooked up to his tiny veins to hydrate him. It was a terrifying time, but Beth finally felt Charlie was going to get the help he needed. She had been labeled as a hysterical mother, so she was asked to stay away from the nurses caring for Charlie. Her behavior, the doctors told her, was interfering with her son's medical care.

When Charlie was released, doctors told Beth that the problem was an allergic reaction to a certain type of virus. Whenever he was exposed to this virus, they said, he would need to go back on the TPN feeding tube. But they insisted he would grow out of this condition by the age of 4.

Beth was as skeptical as she was mystified. She'd never heard of such an allergy and she doubted that Charlie would make such a dramatic turnaround in less than three years. But she began an intense Web-based research project to learn all she could about virus allergies. Oddly, she found nothing online that explained anything related to Charlie's condition. Meanwhile he was getting worse.

Perhaps if she could review Charlie's medical records, Beth thought, she could find something that would give her a clue about what was going on. But when Beth contacted the doctor's office, the staff refused to give her the records. She spoke to several members of the doctor's team, eventually reaching the doctor himself, in her attempt to get a copy of Charlie's files.

"Why do you need these records?" he asked. "You won't understand them anyway. Your son has eosinophilic gastroenteritis. You won't find any information about it anywhere. It's very rare."

Beth's ears perked up. "Wait a minute. What did you say?" The gastroenterologist repeated the words reluctantly. "Spell it for me, slowly," said Beth.

"Don't bother looking it up on the Internet," cautioned the doctor. "There's nothing credible on it."

Beth hung up, tired of being kept out of the loop of her son's care. She went straight to her computer and kicked off what proved to be a fruitful search for resources regarding Charlie's diagnosis. This was back in 2000 when online resources were more difficult to locate, but Beth found a listserv where parents of other children struggling with eosinophilic gastroenteritis (EGE) shared ideas and solutions. This helpful patient/caregiver community led Beth to a huge amount of EGE information as well as referrals to physicians who specialize in treating it. She read medical journal articles about EGE with a medical dictionary at hand, deciphering the vocabulary. When she didn't understand something in the articles, she called her son's pediatrician for an explanation.

After a few months of research, Beth realized several things:

- EGE was a chronic disease, so Charlie would not grow out of it.
- EGE was more common than the family was led to believe.
- There were doctors who treated it as a specialty and they were described by other EGE parents as empathetic, patient and, most importantly, knowledgeable.
- The gastroenterologist she had been dealing with was more interested in proving Beth wrong than finding a solution for Charlie's condition.

Beth and her husband returned to the gastroenterologist's office, armed with numerous articles and answers.

"How do you know that Charlie will outgrow EGE?" she asked.

"Well, most children outgrow it," the doctor replied.

"'Most children' means nothing to me. What if he doesn't? What then?"

Beth refused to be dismissed, and demanded a plan for her child.

Beth was no longer willing to be passive about her son's care. She was his primary advocate, an active member of his team, well-versed in his condition and needed to be treated as such. She insisted that any doctor treating Charlie must be experienced in his disease category *and* willing to acknowledge her as an empowered, informed caregiver.

Beth and her husband fired that gastroenterologist and began taking Charlie to physicians recommended by other EGE parents. They have since received the targeted care they sought and which Charlie required.

Beth also soon joined forces with a handful of other parents to form the American Partnership for Eosinophilic Disorders (APFED, at www.apfed.org), which received its 501c3 status as a non-profit organization in 2002. APFED has since grown to become the leading resource for families and physicians involved in EGE, wielding a strong legislative influence and hosting regular conferences for doctors who treat the condition and families touched by it.

Charlie's condition is now managed by medications and therapies administered by health care professionals familiar with the unique characteristics of EGE. His family's difficult but inspiring experience illustrates the value of putting a name to a condition and conducting thorough research. It also demonstrates how empowerment can do more than improve doctor-patient communications; it can save a life.

A STEP-BY-STEP GUIDE

The following tips should help you navigate your first steps toward patient empowerment:

1. IDENTIFY YOUR DIAGNOSIS

First and foremost, you must get a clear and detailed definition of your diagnosis. This is what I call "finding the what." You want to make sure you arm yourself with the accurate name for what the physician says you are dealing with, even if it means asking your doctor to repeat things a few times. You'll discover nothing but frustration by heading down the wrong path if you begin researching the wrong thing.

Search for "breast cancer" and you will have to plod through millions of sites that the search engine deems relevant to your query. But a search for the phrase "HER-2/neu type breast cancer" returns far fewer links. Add "premenopausal" to this same string of words and the number of results shrinks dramatically.

Insider's Tip:

The more specific your search, the more specific the Internet will be.

This same recommendation applies in the prediagnosis stage. If you have symptoms that worry you, and you want to conduct online research before you see a doctor, be careful about how you dive into that process. Entering such vague terms as "fatigue" or "headache" into a search engine will return way too many links, none of which will be helpful. These general symptoms are common in numerous innocent and correctible patterns (too much caffeine, perhaps) as well as life-threatening conditions (brain tumor, for one). Online research that is broad and non-specific will drown you in a sea of confusion and fear.

When we're worried about our health, we usually assume the worst. And the worst of the worst is readily available online. Don't make the mistake of placing yourself in a dangerous category without first getting confirmation from a physician so you can conduct a more informed search.

2. DETERMINE HOW YOUR DIAGNOSIS IS UNIQUE
TO YOU

I cannot emphasize this point enough. Even if you know your precise form of a disease, there are numerous factors that make your clinical situation different from that of another person who receives the exact same diagnosis. Your body chemistry, your age, your overall health, the stage at which your disease was caught, the distinct biology of your cells, your family history, even environmental factors in your region all contribute to what makes your case unique. Not all cancers or conditions that fall under the same label behave in the same ways.

All of this means that when you research your condition online, you must remember that what works for you might not be what works for another patient, and vice versa. In addition – and this is critical – when you review online statistics, remember that they are only statistics. Keep them in perspective. Statistics reflect the broad range of patient stories and outcomes, and may differ greatly from what you experience.

Insider's Tip:

Remember that statistics reflect large generalities. They are only helpful when they apply to your specific situation. You are a patient, not a statistic.

Remember that medical research moves quickly and new treatment options are becoming available all the time, so some websites do not contain the latest data. So use the Internet to become informed, but remember that your case is yours alone.

3. MAINTAIN A BIT OF SKEPTICISM

We like to believe that the medical system and the people who run it are infallible. Unfortunately, health care professionals are human and medical science is flawed.

As a patient, you must balance trust with skepticism because errors can arise.

In most cases, mistakes are minimal and don't cause problems. In others, they can lead to major issues for patients.

For example, if your physician orders blood tests and the results reveal a serious condition that requires immediate treatment, then you want to make sure the results are yours and not someone else's. This is why specialists often repeat the same tests that family practitioners have already run.

The same rule applies when you begin online research about your condition. As you review individual sites and read up on what you have, remember to take what you find with a grain of salt. Listen to your instincts to guide you toward legitimate content. When it comes to your health and survival, skepticism is a beneficial form of resourcefulness.

4. KNOW YOUR OPTIONS

Reliable test results and a definitive diagnosis will help you figure out what your options are. The Internet will widen your perspective past your local doctor and medical facility to see if additional treatments and experts are available. When you have information on what you believe to be credible and reasonable alternatives, you can present these ideas to your physician to get an expert's perspective.

When I was first diagnosed with chronic lymphocytic leukemia, the local cancer specialists clearly instructed me to begin treatment immediately using the standard therapy applied to most patients with my form of the disease. But the community of patients with whom I had connected through the CLL listserv urged me to seek a second opinion. They led me directly to Dr. Keating at M. D. Anderson. When I saw Dr. Keating and he ran additional tests, he determined that I did not need immediate treatment. If it had not been for those experienced, empowered patients, I would never have known to pursue Keating and would not have benefited from his experimental treatment.

5. Consider the roles of your team members

As you broaden your awareness of your disease category and your unique condition, it's important that you understand the interplay among the various medical experts on your case. Familiarizing yourself with the different roles of generalists vs. specialists will assist you as you do your research and will clarify which questions to bring up with which team members.

I like to think of the highly specialized expert (Dr. Keating, in my case) as the architect of a patient's health care efforts. The architect possesses the vision of what the condition is and can see all treatment possibilities. He or she must be up to speed on the latest "materials" with which to rebuild a person's health. The architect provides the blueprint and then allows others to follow that plan.

The less specialized physicians who administer the treatment plan can be considered the builders. Their expertise and attention to detail is invaluable, but they follow the architect's plan throughout the project.

Insider's Tip:

Find out who does what on your health care team. It will help you keep your perspective on what you learn from each of your doctors.

6. FACTOR IN FAMILY HISTORY

To help you zero in on the proper and most empowering online information, you'll need to know your family history, particularly with regard to your specific condition. A symptom that worries you becomes more significant — and more relevant to your doctor — if it reflects a genetic pattern. (Stomach ache, for example, is an innocent sign of indigestion for most people, but an important symptom to investigate for those with a family history of celiac disease where gluten in bread and other foods inflames the digestive tract.)

During your online research, keep your findings in the proper familial context. Pay particular attention when clinical data relates a condition to the genetic predispositions of certain clinical categories (such as heart disease, specific cancers, stroke, diabetes, high blood pressure, etc.).

7. STAY ON TOP OF YOUR OWN RECORDS

To get a clear understanding of what you're dealing with, it's crucial to organize the data that you gather, as well as all of your own medical records. (This topic is addressed in detail in Chapter Nine.) Create a virtual file on your computer or a hard copy binder and separate it into categories containing the findings of your own research, copies of any reference materials you receive from your doctor, copies of as many lab and test results as possible, copies of all imaging you have done (x-rays, MRIs, CT scans, etc.) and any accompanying reports.

Maintaining your own records will provide a single hub for all your case information that will serve you well as you embark on this journey. The unfortunate reality is that records get lost and misfiled in clinical settings, so you can always provide a back-up copy if that happens to you. As you seek input within online communities focused on your disease category, people will ask about your results on certain tests in order to provide recommendations. They'll be at your fingertips.

With direct access to your medical files, you are better equipped to serve as your own patient advocate.

8. REMEMBER THE EVER-CHANGING NATURE OF THE INTERNET

The Internet is in a constant state of change, just like an organic being. It too has a combination of fat and meat. You must wade through the questionable outer layers in order to get to the real substance. You can find your lifeline on the Web, but you must know how to look. You may return to the same places more than once to find what you need. Your knowledge will expand during your online research, but so will the pertinent content regarding your condition. Be diligent, be patient and be discriminating.

{ Two }

STRENGTHENING YOUR COPING SKILLS

The Importance of Emotional and Spiritual Empowerment

IN MY EXPERIENCE

I was in a thick fog immediately following my initial leukemia diagnosis. I was confused and fearful, not sure which way to turn for answers. Like many people in similar situations, I wanted concrete assurances that I would be okay in the end. I worried as much for my family as I did for myself. Unfortunately, there was no way to see into the future and know what my outcome would be. My condition had a label, but my fate was a mystery.

Within the first few days, I found myself seeking guidance from a higher authority. I arranged a meeting with David Serkin-Poole, a clergyman and spiritual leader I had known for many years. I hoped David's advice and counsel would help me make sense of the surreal nightmare in which I had landed. It ended up being one of the most important conversations I had during that early phase, since it helped me to embrace the concept of the unknowable.

"It's true, none of us knows what will happen to us," David acknowledged. "But there are other, perhaps more important things that we do know."

David encouraged me to focus less on how much time I had left on this earth, since that was something that was largely out of my control. He recommended that I ponder what I stood for, what my life to that point had meant. He shared with me a wonderful book called *Ethical Wills* by Barry K. Baines, urging me to create such a document for myself. The exercise, he explained, would allow me to express who I was as a person – a man, a husband, a father, a citizen – rather than as a leukemia patient. It would define my beliefs and accomplishments leading up to that point and clarify how I wanted to "behave" as I proceeded into this tunnel of treatments, whatever the eventual outcome.

I was then able to tackle the challenges related to my diagnosis from a stronger place. Most importantly, it opened me up to possibilities and opportunities I might not have otherwise considered. Specifically, when I came across the online community of CLL patients that would prove to be my lifeline, my sense of spiritual empowerment gave me the courage to listen to their input. I believe to this day that following my cantor's advice was one of the most significant early steps in my journey away from cancer.

COMMUNICATING, CONNECTING, COPING

I received valuable support from a spiritual leader whose words and wisdom bolstered me in the early days of my diagnosis. But there are countless alternative ways to seek emotional support as you begin your life as a patient or caregiver facing a serious medical issue.

Wherever you can find sources of strength — from prayer, meditation, yoga, family, community, advocacy or some combination of things that works for you — it is crucial that you seek them out. And the sooner, the bet-

Insider's Tip:

There is no right or wrong way to strengthen your resolve. Design your own wellness program.

ter. Teams of medical professionals will be working on your body's behalf. You must ensure that your emotional self gets the same treatment.

How then does the Internet come into play when it comes to emotional empowerment? Good question, with a surprising number of answers. Here are just a few things the Web can do to help boost emotional and spiritual health:

1. Prove to you that you're not alone.
2. Introduce you to tips and strategies that have helped other people cope.
3. Tell hopeful stories of people with your condition who conquer statistics and beat the odds.

4. Allow you and your family to communicate efficiently with others who want to help.

5. Provide a way for you to keep a journal of your experiences, either for private or public consumption.

6. Delve deeper than mainstream media into the latest information on your condition.

7. Offer an opportunity for you to serve as an advocate for yourself and others.

Your doctor won't be able to measure the effectiveness of your efforts in this regard. There are no lab tests or imaging techniques that can

Insider's Tip:

Emotional wellness is an important component of physical health.

track the fluctuations of emotional health. But nobody can deny the importance of talking to yourself about getting well (as opposed to dwelling on thoughts related to being ill). Focusing on the positive goes a long way in strengthening you at an extremely vulnerable time.

Learn as much as you can about those who have fought this battle before you and drink in the power of their success stories. Tell yourself not only that you are strong enough to handle this, but that you are also strong enough to ask for help when you need it. You might also choose to use the Web as a way to give to others, as there is nothing more powerful than reaching out to someone else.

For individuals battling serious medical crises, the Internet functions as the world's biggest support group. It can provide compassion, energy, efficiency and literally millions of listeners. Using it as a tool for emotional empowerment allows you to focus more clearly on what is most important – conquering your illness.

GETTING AN EARLY START

If you are new to all of this, you may feel in shock as you ponder what you or your loved one is about to undergo. This is a very common and understandable response. But it speaks to the importance of emotional empowerment. During these early days, you will be faced with a lot of new, potentially frightening information. The sturdier your emotional footing, the more you will be able to process on an intellectual level.

For your head to be effective, your heart must be whole. So reach out in whatever direction you need and build yourself a powerful foundation.

SEEKING STRENGTH IN COMMUNITY

The benefits of connecting with online communities are explored in more detail in Chapter Six, but it's also an important subject to address in the context of emotional empowerment.

When I began researching CLL online in 1996, I discovered more than I set out to find. There were already numerous resources available to me and people like me, even given the limitations of the then-youthful Internet. My intent was to gather as much information as I could on my disease and my treatment options. What I found was a CLL listserv that supported a community of fellow patients and caregivers who were dealing with the exact same diagnosis and were at various points along the path of treatment.

Among this group was a man named Charlie Jennings of Seattle.[1] He received his diagnosis at roughly the same

1   Not his real name.

time I did, had a type and progression of leukemia similar to mine and lived near me in the Seattle area. Along with other members of the listserv, Charlie and I began communicating regularly about CLL and how it affected us and our families. Soon those of us who lived close enough to do so decided to meet in person. Charlie was among them.

I looked for the first time at the individuals with whom I had been communicating electronically about this scary disease and I was struck by how normal – even healthy – most of them looked. Not one of them appeared to have what we had all been told was a terminal illness. The online fellowship was enormously empowering to me; seeing first-hand that CLL patients were living normal lives was an unexpected bonus.

Charlie was the one whom I was most excited to meet since our clinical profiles were so similar. He did not disappoint. Healthy and hearty, he was living, breathing proof that there was hope.

"In the beginning, the connections I made on the Internet were a big help to me," says Charlie, looking back at those early days. "When I was diagnosed, I thought I was going to die. The doctors said the 'c' word – cancer – and told me it's incurable. I thought I would have several years of life and then be out," he recalls. More than a decade later, Charlie's leukemia has still never reared its head beyond the occasional elevated white blood cell count. He has never had any problem or required any treatment.

Charlie's and my shared experience illustrates the ways in which reaching out to fellow "sufferers" can have enormously valuable effects. Finding out that you're not alone in this can be hugely therapeutic. Some people might want to sit back and observe online discussions; others might find themselves taking more active roles. There is no right or wrong way. The key is to tap into the resources available to you so that you can take what you need from them. Someone out there has been where you are, felt what you feel and feared what you fear. Find them or their stories and learn how they picked themselves up off of the floor and moved forward.

REACHING OUT SO OTHERS CAN HELP

Brain cancer was not in Jill Peterson's plans. This mother of three young kids got the news at the age of 43 that would change her life and the lives of those around her. Although she exhibited strength and determination throughout her various courses of treatment, she struggled with how to juggle the demands of her illness alongside those of daily family life.

A resourceful co-worker of Jill's husband came up with a solution that supported everyone concerned, including friends and loved ones who wanted desperately to help but did not know how. He set up a simple website with an interactive calendar function that allowed people to volunteer to deliver meals and/or drive Jill to radiation treatments on specified days.

"I was just too ill at that time to take care of myself," Jill recalls. "So five days a week, I had people stepping forward and bringing me to my treatments. And there were days, I kid you not, where I wouldn't have gotten out of bed except for the fact that my doorbell would usually ring at about 9:15

in the morning with somebody standing there out of the goodness of their heart saying, 'Are you ready to go?' And they would drive me to my treatment, sit and wait for me in the waiting room, then drive me home."

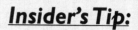

Insider's Tip:

Be open to people's desire to help. It will benefit you and them.

A simple online scheduling tool got Jill to her appointments, put food on her family's table and gave those who cared an opportunity to ease her burden.

"I could not have done it without the love and care of my community," Jill declares. "And I never knew the community was as big as it was."

As the Web evolves, an increasing number of tools are available that can help in times of medical crisis. This list offers just a sampling of the numerous ways you can use the Internet to help others help you and your family:

- **Caring Bridge (www.caringbridge.org)** Free, personalized websites that support and connect loved ones during critical illness, treatment and recovery.

- **CarePages** (**www.carepages.com**) Free patient blogs that connect friends and family during a health challenge.

- **Blogger** (**www.blogger.com**) Free blogging tools and templates.

- **Facebook** (**www.facebook.com**) The popular social networking site offers quick and easy communication to broad groups of people.

- **Twitter** (**www.twitter.com**) Disseminate brief updates quickly and easily to key members of your circle.

- **LotsaHelpingHands** (**www.lotsahelpinghands. com**) Tools that help individuals assist anyone who needs support due to illness, infirmity, financial need, military leave, etc.

GOING BEYOND AVAILABLE MEDIA

When traditional patient education materials and mainstream media fail to provide the support that patients seek, the Internet can serve as a new frontier. Used responsibly, the Web gives patients a voice and presents new opportunities for empowerment where none previously existed.

That was the case when Lynne Matallana finally received a diagnosis to explain her chronic pain after a frustrating odyssey on which she sought the expertise of 37 physicians. Eventually Lynne learned that she had fibromyalgia, a condition unknown to her or anyone she knew. Her diagnosis came in the early 1990s, pre-Internet, at which point Lynne sought information from books, magazine articles and anecdotal reports. As the Web emerged, Lynne gradually connected with others who battled the same or similar illnesses with chronic pain. Even as the online fibromyalgia community grew, there continued to be a startling lack of useful patient education resources.

"I spent almost two and a half years in bed not knowing exactly what was wrong with me, being misdiagnosed with lupus and MS and psychiatric problems and just about everything that you could possibly imagine," Lynne remembers. "I used to sit there and think, okay, if I ever get to the point where I am better, I am going to try to do something that will help other people not have to go through the hell that I went through during that time period."

Insider's Tip:

Use the Web as a blank canvas. Use the tools you prefer to create your own forms of interconnectedness.

Lynne's background in marketing and public relations meant that she knew how to communicate on a grand scale, so she began to think about the value of raising fibromyalgia awareness.

"I wanted to let people know that there were a lot of people like myself whom I found on the Internet, who were going from doctor to doctor and were basically being told that there was nothing wrong with them; that this was just all psychological and in their head," she says. "But we all knew that that wasn't the case. We knew that there was something physiological going on within our bodies."

After finally getting her diagnosis, Lynne partnered with Karen Lee Richards, another patient whom she met online, to form the National Fibromyalgia Association (www.

fmaware.org). What began as a quest for information has grown into the life work of these two resourceful and empowered women.

Lynne's story is an example of how the Internet can start where traditional media stop. When people are hungry for patient-driven support and content, the Web has filled a tremendous gap. The Web offers endless opportunities for self-empowerment when people desire to do more to help themselves.

SHARING YOUR STORY

Like Lynne Matallana, Matthew Zachary felt alone in his diagnosis. As a talented 21-year-old concert pianist with a promising future, Matthew received devastating news: brain cancer. While doctors went to work treating him, Matthew got busy trying to learn more about his condition and what others in his situation were doing to cope. He quickly realized the gigantic gap in resources related to cancers in young adults. Numerous websites and support groups focused on cases affecting either pediatric or older adult populations, but none was devoted to his demographic.

"I felt very isolated," Matt recalls. "There was no real support group for people my age. I was invited to several 'sit in a circle and share your stories' events and everyone there was at least 20 or 30 years older than I was."

Matt struggled to find any information he could as his treatments continued and he finally emerged from his ordeal cancer-free. However, he was forced to modify his musical aspirations due to diminished fine motor function in his hands. He pursued a career in advertising and Web development instead. His exposure to online marketing would lead him to his new professional calling: advocacy.

"I developed a vested interest in understanding what cancer advocacy meant and came to the conclusion that it was all about ensuring the next 'me' wouldn't have to go through the same injustices that I did," Matt explains. "I learned that survival rates and quality of life for young adults with cancer had not improved in 30 years. That was the spark I needed to dive right into this fight head first."

Insider's Tip:

Consider advocacy as a way to shift your focus toward the larger fight against a disease rather than your individual struggle with it.

Matt's motivation to give back to his peers led him to his advocacy role. He founded the I'm Too Young For This! Cancer Foundation (http://i2y.com) in 2007, which is now the nation's leading grassroots advocate for young adults affected by what Matt describes as "stupid cancer." From there, Matt and his colleagues took to the "webwaves" to give a voice to the movement. The "Stupid Cancer Show" talk-radio broadcast airs live every week on the Internet and is syndicated internationally to more than 25,000 listeners.

"I feel it's really driven change in the sense that young adult survivorship is now something that's part of a global dialogue," Matt says. "We think the establishment is now really taking notice and I'm very happy to have been a part of helping to make that happen."

WHAT WORKS FOR YOU?

When you're feeling crushed by the enormity of a frightening diagnosis, one of the best things you can do for yourself right away is to hone your coping skills. Start with the basic techniques that have proven effective for you in the past. Then consider the Internet. You may be surprised by its comforting qualities and how that online community can help steel you for whatever is to come.

{ THREE }

IDENTIFYING YOUR OWN OPERATING SYSTEM

How Do You Seek and Process Information?

IN MY EXPERIENCE

When my second blood test confirmed my doctor's suspicions, I knew I needed to learn all I could about chronic lymphocytic leukemia. As a medical journalist, I had some professional insight into how to research and report on conditions. But I was a complete novice as a patient. My fear and anxiety didn't help matters much either.

I sensed that I could find helpful information on the Internet, still a brand new tool, but I was unsure how best to undertake such a search. Even if I were able to locate anything applicable, I was not in the best emotional state to process what I might find.

Our neighbor and tech-savvy friend David Nudelman heard through the grapevine about my diagnosis and came to the rescue immediately. That first night, he arrived at our home, rolled up his sleeves and sat down at my computer. Esther and I watched as he navigated through what was a far less user-friendly technological landscape to find information and resources that I could use. He quickly found the CLL listserv that would eventually lead me to Houston and the doctors who have guided my treatment to this day.

The most important aspect of David's assistance was his ability to foster those life-changing connections for me in a way that was efficient but detached. I was overwrought; using David as a filter in the initial hours of my life as a cancer patient made all the difference. Had I been the one wading through leukemia statistics, the data would have likely knocked me off my chair. I needed him to open the appropriate door so that I could cross the threshold in my own time and on my own terms.

MANAGED CHAOS

By reading this book, you have already demonstrated your interest in becoming more empowered. If your next stop is the Internet, where information comes at you as if it's being shot out of a fire hose, it's important for you to figure out how best to receive that onslaught. You need to determine the best ways for you to seek and process the available data.

When it comes to health resources, the Internet has it all – the good, the bad and the ugly. It ranges from the most basic (definitions and terms) to the moderately complicated (online debates surrounding the best courses of action) to the extremely complex (technical papers intended for clinical audiences). You'll find a nearly endless supply of information. The question is: What is the best way for you to tackle it?

Insider's Tip:

Think back to when you were a full-time student and try to recall what researching techniques worked best for you then. You can modify those same approaches and apply them to your current quest.

There is no right or wrong way to search for online information related to your condition. Spending a little time "interviewing" yourself at the outset will save you enormous amounts of wasted energy when you'll already be stretched fairly thin.

Ask yourself the following questions:

1. Do you want to ease into your education about your condition or would you prefer to dive in and gather as much data as you can as quickly as possible?

2. When it comes to online communities for those who share your condition, would you prefer to sit back and observe or become an actively involved member of discussions and debates?

3. Do you prefer to work alone or would you like a research partner by your side?

4. Do you absorb information better when it is in written or audio or video form?

5. Do you thirst for high-level, scientific information? Do you want to review sources that are written for the lay or professional audience? Or both?

6. If English is not your first language, would you be more comfortable searching for online resources that are posted in your native tongue?

Your ability to learn and participate via the Web will evolve over time as you become more accustomed to "patienthood" and more familiar with what you're dealing with. This was certainly true for me. I began my journey as a "lurker" on the CLL listserv, observing from an invisible position, which was where I was comfortable at that point. As I became less afraid and more empowered, I started to participate more and more. I later became a vocal member of the online CLL community and helped draw tentative newcomers into the group.

Conducting research on the Internet is like sitting down to an exotic meal. You begin with small bites to see what you like then you gradually get used to what is being served and open yourself up to new dishes and larger portions. Certain things may not appeal to you, but you respond favorably to other offerings. You and your appetite are yours alone, and you should approach this new experience in the way that turns out to be the most satisfying – and fruitful – for you.

Insider's Tip:

Don't put additional pressure on yourself by assuming that you're not smart enough to absorb medical information. Conduct your research in the manner that suits you best. It will make you feel more – not less – confident.

WHICH TYPE ARE YOU?

Here are just a few profiles of information-seeking styles:

The Hunter/Gatherer

This proactive person wants to find any and all resources related to his condition as soon as humanly possible. The more information he can gather, the more empowered he feels. He sits right down at his computer as soon as he feels capable and gets to work becoming an active member of his own team.

Mike McKelheer fit into this category once he got over his initial shock. Following a routine physical in 2007, this active, physically fit 67-year-old got the surprising diagnosis of prostate cancer. It took him a few days to overcome his instinct to run and hide. ("I got the news on a Friday and I was shaking like a leaf all of Friday and Saturday," he says.) But once he felt up to it, he took control.

"My son sat down with me and said, 'Dad you can't do anything about it. It's there and now we've got to deal with it.' So here's my son telling me to grow up," he remembers. "So I got on the Internet and went to the library and a few bookstores and bought everything I possibly could buy on prostate cancer. It was quite helpful."

Mike also sought out other men who had dealt with prostate cancer. "I wanted to call them. I wanted to talk to them," he says.

His dedication proved invaluable, as it led him to groundbreaking technology being developed in his own region. "I heard about (this new treatment option) and started researching it and kind of zoned in on it," Mike explains. He asked his physicians if such an option would be suitable for him, and they got involved in the conversation. Mike ended up being the first patient to use the company's technology, which acts as a GPS system for radiation treatment of prostate cancer.

Mike's subsequent radiation therapy was successful and he never slowed the pace of his active routine. "I never balked or changed my lifestyle during the whole ordeal," he says. "While I was receiving my shots and going through radiation, I worked full time with no missed days. I worked out three nights a week and went snow skiing and water skiing and hiking into lakes to fly fish. All of this helped put my mind at ease.

"It's really up to you," Mike adds. "You listen to all the doctors and you pick out little things from each one of them, but now you've got more options. I think I made the right decision. I want to be skiing when I'm a hundred years old."

The Partner

This patient prefers to have someone else absorb, process and respond to the mountain of information related to her condition. She is prepared to take an active role in her own case, but does best when she has someone by her side serving as research facilitator.

Patricia Beck had her husband, Rob, serve as intermediary during her struggle with soft tissue sarcoma. When they first received her diagnosis, Patricia and Rob faced it head-on, although she recalls vividly the fear she felt in the beginning.

"It's terribly frightening," Patricia says. "I guess my first emotion was just to be really scared, and then sadness kicks in pretty quick and a little anxiety and a whole lot of negative feelings. But I think I pretty quickly put my faith in the doctors and my family to help me through it. I also prayed continuously throughout our medical journey."

At the helm of the family ship was Rob, who immediately assumed the role of case manager on Patricia's behalf. "I'm a numbers guy and one of those typical 'fix it' type guys," Rob admits. "I kept a notebook and records on everything that we did, everything that the doctors said, the medications she was on and all of that."

Documenting the details of his wife's condition and treatment gave Rob (and, in turn, Patricia) a greater sense of empowerment and helped them better understand the doctors' recommendations. "It was so obvious to me that all of those guys talked and that there was great continuity. They knew what was going on, and we knew what was going on. This continuity made us feel pretty comfortable," reports Rob.

When Patricia looks back on her illness, she credits others who helped her through. "I had so much support from family and friends that it was just wonderful," she says.

The Trusting Patient

This individual worries about becoming overwhelmed by the abundance of information he might find about his condition and his prognosis and prefers to leave the clinical research up to the scientists and the medical decisions up to the physicians. His job, he feels, is to find the best doctors for his illness, connect with them, and then let them do their jobs. For some patients, that means conducting online research to find the experts in the field. For others, it means trusting that the medical team assigned to the case is at the top of their game.

This was the philosophy of Ed Edwards, a career firefighter whose advanced lung cancer was discovered while he was enjoying his retirement. After Ed coughed up a small amount of blood one day, his family doctor x-rayed his chest and found a tumor.

"Luckily my doctor was already plugged into the local university hospital's system," Ed says. He had a CAT scan almost immediately and within a week had an appointment with a member of the university medical center's "dream team" of lung cancer specialists who work together coordinating a patient's care.

"I didn't realize it at the time, but having a team made it a lot easier," Ed reports. "As I became a little bit sicker and weaker, my desire to make decisions and my ability to analyze things wasn't quite as good. So having already been part of this team, the decisions were basically made. I was given the options and was already plugged in, so it made life much easier not only for me but for my wife because we already had the confidence in the group. They had a plan."

That plan saved Ed's life and helped him and his loved ones face the situation with confidence. "The plan was laid out pretty much from the beginning, and it just took that anxiety away for me and my family," he says.

The High-Level Processor

This person is more than comfortable diving into highly technical materials related to health conditions even when she possesses no formal medical training. The more complex the references, the more empowered she feels. For her, the Internet is a gold mine of clinical papers and research study data. Those who seek this level of information can learn of the latest breakthroughs at the same time as the leading physicians.

The high-level processor will find a wealth of information on websites that cater to the health care professional audience (as opposed to patients). Medscape.com, MedPageToday.com and eMedicine.com are among the sites that deliver educational and news-related content to physicians but are open to public viewing. Medical societies also offer technical content related to their specialties and consumers are free to browse their pages. The American Society of Hematology (for doctors specializing in leukemia or lymphoma), the American College of Cardiology (heart disease) and the American College of Rheumatology (arthritis) are just a few examples of these clinical specialty websites.

Gretchen Cover was diagnosed with chronic lymphocytic leukemia in 1998 at a time when her Internet use, like many people's, was essentially limited to email. When she and her family moved to a small town several states away from the Johns Hopkins team originally treating her, Gretchen began increasing her online activity. "That's when the Internet became critical because I became a support group of one," she remembers.

Since then, Gretchen has become: 1) An active member of the online CLL community, serving as a list manager for the CLL list for the Association of Cancer Online Resources (ACOR), and 2) Someone who easily digests clinical materials related to her disease.

"My level of sophistication when it comes to processing this stuff has ramped up 1000 percent since I got started," she says. "I don't know how to read a CBC (complete blood count), but I know how to find the information I need and to diplomatically relay information to the various doctors I need to get it to. I'm very comfortable in the clinical realm and I use the Internet as an advocacy tool."

She is quick to emphasize the need for patients to use what they find to create productive dialogue with physicians. "Too many patients read things and use it to challenge or second guess their doctors, which has no value or consequence," she warns. "If what you find pertains to your case and would advance diagnosis, treatment or knowledge, then that can be helpful.

But don't quiz your doctors to see if they're on top of things."

The Internet, Gretchen believes, teaches us the importance of second opinions. "You don't have to understand everything you read online, but you'll start seeing the same doctors' names and clinics over and over," she explains. "If you can't go to them in person, you should encourage your doctor to get in touch with them because most experts are willing to work with other doctors. Just remember that you and your doctor are partners and you have to keep that going. Use what you find to further, not challenge, the relationship or it could be detrimental to your health."

The Lay-Level Processor

Sometimes it's more comfortable and less frightening to approach a medical condition more gingerly, limiting yourself to information that is intentionally simplified for the lay audience. If this describes you, there are endless resources available online to help answer your questions. The bulk of the Internet's patient information is presented in an easy-to-understand language so that it can be consumed by a wide variety of non-technical researchers.

A NOTE ON PRIVACY

The advent of the Internet has introduced new concerns about maintaining and protecting the privacy of its users. When you begin searching for online information related to a personal medical condition, these concerns may be at the top of your mind.

While you should use common sense when it comes to your activities on the Web, don't let your desire for anonymity prevent you from diving into whatever resources you can find. There are plenty of ways to find what you need without divulging your identity or your personal health information, unless you want to do so.

Remember that every patient who explores the Internet in search of answers and support is in the exact same position as you and also has an interest in privacy. Since diseases do not discriminate, there are plenty of people whose real names are recognizable (celebrities, politicians, etc.) and simply use aliases when they engage in online discourse.

There are sites on the Web that allow people to find community while still remaining anonymous and invisible. One of the most interesting is Second Life (www.secondlife. com), where patients can sign on *using only their virtual identities* to forums dedicated to discussion and debate about given medical conditions. Such digital destinations – and their shroud of anonymity – offer opportunities for social relationships and information-exchange among individuals who might not otherwise pursue them.

CHANGING HABITS

The most important aspect of identifying what type of information-seeker you are is figuring out your initial comfort level. That will likely change quite dramatically over the course of your experience as a patient or caregiver.

First, it is extremely common to feel overwhelmed and under-informed at the beginning of your new situation. Facing endless amounts of Web-based information and figuring out

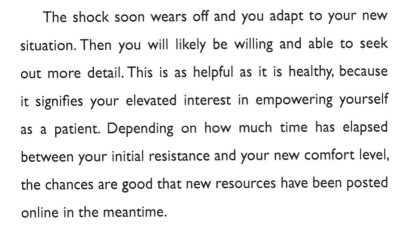

Insider's Tip:

There's nothing wrong with starting slowly. Your pace will increase as you become more informed.

how it applies to you can be daunting at best and paralyzing at worst. In the early stage, people tend to tiptoe into the information-gathering process.

The shock soon wears off and you adapt to your new situation. Then you will likely be willing and able to seek out more detail. This is as helpful as it is healthy, because it signifies your elevated interest in empowering yourself as a patient. Depending on how much time has elapsed between your initial resistance and your new comfort level, the chances are good that new resources have been posted online in the meantime.

Adjusting your information-seeking habits and returning to the Internet over time offers these advantages:

1. Your emotional strength will solidify as you travel down this path and you will likely be open to things

now that you did not feel you could handle when you were first diagnosed.

2. New materials and resources are constantly added to the Internet, so what you find now might be more relevant and useful than just a few months ago.

3. Your health situation will change as you progress through treatment, so you'll benefit from new categories of information at different points along your journey.

THE PARENT TRAP

Perhaps more than anyone else, parents of children diagnosed with serious conditions are desperate for answers. Mothers and fathers scramble to find any applicable resources that might lead toward healthy outcomes. But this emotionally charged quest can be more frustrating than productive if parents don't first identify the ways in which they can process what they find.

I've observed numerous situations in which parents became disproportionately influenced by the *first* things they read or heard about the condition their family was facing, even when it came from a medical professional. If that first bit of information is negative, ominous or insufficient, it can set a tone that jolts the entire endeavor off-track at the outset. Seeking second opinions that could lead to more hopeful results is perhaps more important for parents of sick children than it is for adult patients.

Portland, Oregon resident Karen Reynolds' nightmare started when her son, Cooper, began having terrible headaches as a 6-year-old. Their pediatrician helped identify the cause: a right-side brain mass that needed to be surgically removed. But when the surgeons finished their work, they reported disappointing news. "They were only able to remove about 35 percent of it and they kind of just sent us on our way," Karen remembers. "I wasn't real comfortable with that. I felt like we needed a really good team to back us up." Cooper's problems were exacerbated by a new seizure disorder, which caused up to six seizures every day immediately following the first surgery.

So Karen went to work doing her own research to learn more about the family's options. She reached out online to other parents, the Epilepsy Foundation, the Epilepsy Society and the Brain Tumor Foundation. "I couldn't get off of the Internet," she says. "I was constantly looking up anything I could possibly find trying to educate myself on what we were going to do, what we were looking at. Because I truly believed that we were the ones who were going to have to dictate where this was going."

Her search was fruitful, leading the family to a nearby pediatric neuro-oncologist who soon was heading up what Karen refers to as "Team Cooper." The team also featured a pediatric neurosurgeon, a neuro-psychiatrist and numerous supporting health care professionals. The team performed a second surgery, in which they were able to remove 95 percent of the remaining tumor, which dramatically decreased Cooper's seizures and helped return him to his old self.

For Karen, the key was seeking a second opinion, even after her child's first surgery, because she could see that he was still unwell. "Getting on the Internet is very important," she emphasizes. "A lot of parents communicate that way back and forth, you can read blogs, the Epilepsy Society has a wonderful website and most of the hospitals have websites. I would not be scared of second opinions by any stretch of the imagination. It was a great day to stand in that ICU and have all those wonderful doctors who became our angels standing there looking at my son, who walked out the next day and went home."

A STYLE ALL YOUR OWN

The Internet shoots a huge supply of information at you, which can make you feel as if you have no control. You may feel like you are drowning in data, unsure what is useful and what isn't. Your job as an empowered patient is to identify the ways in which you can most effectively and efficiently process what the Web will send your way. You'll be better able to benefit from its wealth of resources if you ponder your learning patterns and pace yourself. Empowered patients know how to balance the wisdom of the medical professionals with the insight and experience of the global patient community on the Web.

{ Four }

Finding the Experts

Get Help from the Right People, Places and Patients

In my experience

On the evening of my initial diagnosis, I began my journey toward the proper physician, facility and treatment. With the help of our friend David Nudelman, I signed up for the leukemia listserv via ACOR (the Association of Cancer Online Resources at www.acor.org). Although the ACOR site was new, it offered the same important service it provides today: bundling emails within various disease-specific communities and distributing them to individuals who have joined one of the ACOR groups. Most significantly, ACOR offers sufficient connectivity for people who need — as I did that night — to engage in whatever dialog is taking place regarding a particular type of disease.

I immediately began corresponding with one of the ACOR leukemia community's most vocal patient leaders, Barbara "GrannyBarb" Lackritz from St. Louis. As a veteran patient, she knew exactly how to provide the two most important things I needed at that point: 1) reassurance to calm my fears and 2) experience to guide me to a specialist in chronic lymphocytic leukemia. With her help, we identified one of the nation's "top docs" in CLL at that time: Dr. Michael Keating, based at the University of Texas M.D. Anderson Cancer Center in Houston. According to our online research, he was recognized as a CLL clinical leader by the medical community and was well regarded by the patient community. His name popped up frequently in discussions and references related to CLL; he was not simply included in the sponsored lists of "America's Best Doctors" or among the top advertisers on the search engines. In the CLL world, Keating was the real deal.

With the blessing of my local oncologist, I took a trip to see Dr. Keating in Texas. Given his familiarity with CLL, he recommended a course of treatment for me that combined a less aggressive early phase followed by an experimental approach (via a clinical trial) as my disease progressed. He gave me the courage to face my cancer. He gave Esther and me confidence that I would likely be around for many years to come.

Careful research and utilizing the expertise of patient advocates led me to the doctor, the facility and the treatment that best suited my particular condition.

LEARNING FROM THE WISDOM OF OTHERS

Once you have received your diagnosis, you must balance the expertise of your existing physician(s) with a healthy dose of self-advocacy. Empowering yourself with information beyond what you learn in the doctor's office does not mean that you are challenging that person's proficiency. It is a way to strengthen yourself as a patient so you can better understand your own situation and work in partnership with your entire health care team.

The most important part of your online detective work at this stage of the game is to determine:

1. <u>The doctors</u> who are at the cutting edge for your specific condition.
2. <u>The medical facilities</u> where patients with your condition are having the best outcomes.
3. <u>The patient mentors</u> who have journeyed down this road and are poised to share their knowledge with you.

Although your local doctor is undoubtedly concerned about returning you to health and wellness, he or she is not likely exclusively devoted to your condition. You want to find the doctors and scientists who are leading the fight against your specific form of your disease and benefit from their immersion in that science. If necessary, you may need to go to the facilities where they practice. (Alternatively, you might arrange a remote consultation, which we will discuss in more detail later in this chapter.) Once you have the clinical leaders on your team, you and your local doctor are better set up for decision-making and action.

Insider's Tip:

Seeking a specialist doesn't mean you're abandoning your local doctor. It means you're adding to your health care team, which can also enhance your local doctor's knowledge.

THE HOT SHOT DOCTORS

Jennifer Ambrose was only 34, married with a young son, when a laparoscopic appendectomy revealed a malignant tumor. It was diagnosed as a rare condition known as pseudomyxoma peritoneal cancer. Her local doctors explained the details to Jennifer, including the fact that the mucus created by the tumor had covered her intestinal organs. She decided she needed more information.

"I became consumed by the computer," she reports. Through her research, she learned that among the top specialists in her condition were two near her home in the Midwest. "So I contacted them first," she says. But she was not satisfied with their responses, so she returned to her research in order to cast her net a bit wider. She contacted the physician whose name appeared throughout the Web pages that she had visited. He practiced on the West Coast, but she called his office and told his assistant she would be willing to pay for his time to review her case and consult with her over the phone.

He called Jennifer soon after she sent her records. "He told me he had looked at my pictures and asked me what I would like to know," she says. "He spent a good half hour with me on the phone and addressed all my questions with answers that were beyond what I needed. And as soon as I hung up the telephone, I said to my husband, 'We're going to California to meet this guy.' The sound of his voice, his knowledge – it was just too perfect."

Four months after her diagnosis, Jennifer flew with her family to California and underwent a nine-hour surgery led by the physician she found online. He determined the best course of action for her and used state-of-the-art surgical and follow-up chemotherapy procedures that had proven effective for metastasized abdominal cancers – even one as rare as hers.

Jennifer is now cancer-free and credits her recovery to that surgeon, whom she located online and contacted directly. "I'm almost thankful it happened because it reaffirmed the importance of so many things in my life, like my husband and my son and my family," she says. In fact, just two months after her surgery and chemo, Jennifer became pregnant with her second child.

Jennifer is living proof of the effectiveness of online patient empowerment. She learned that the physicians who know most about a condition will be those whose names pop up most frequently during research. They are the authors of the clinical papers, the doctors mentioned by patients posting to the listservs and the leaders of clinical trials. These are the gurus, the national experts, the people you want on your side.

So how do you go about finding them, screening them and reaching out to them as Jennifer did? Follow these tips:

Remember names

Keep a notepad by your computer as you search websites related to your disease, symptoms, diagnostic tests, treatments and patient communities. Watch for repeated references to the same physician. The names that keep recurring are often the smartest minds in the business and you want them pondering your condition. Some will be physicians in clinical practice, some will teach at medical schools and others will be researchers. Create a roster of these leaders, along with notes detailing as much information as you can about them (including links to the websites where you saw their names).

Dig into credentials

Once you have a list of experts in your condition, begin learning all you can about their professional profiles. Are they affiliated with top medical centers or prestigious university hospitals? Have they authored scientific or clinical papers on the subject of your disease? Do they speak to medical audiences at national conferences? Do they get quoted in news articles on the subject of the disease? Another way to "check up" on a doctor is to search through the listings at Vitals.com or BestDoctors. com, both of which offer detailed information on health care professionals.

Look for patient education content

Many of the biggest names in the treatment of an illness appear on webcasts and other programs in which
they speak to patients just like you. In most cases the
top experts thrive on educating patients. They recognize
that local doctors may not be totally up to speed on the
latest discoveries and breakthroughs for each and every
disease, so they devote time to spreading the word. By
spending an hour on a webcast, you just might learn
enough from one of those "gurus" to help you choose
the best treatments and strategies for your disease.

Listen to chatter

The patients who have come before you can serve as
valuable resources when it comes to identifying who's
who among the top doctors in your disease category.
Patients posting to listservs are not typically shy about
expressing their opinions, so listen to what they're saying. If they mention the physicians you've zeroed in on,
have they had positive patient experiences? Have they
felt in better hands? Do they report on their rates of
recovery? These anecdotal comments are worth their

weight in gold because they are unscripted and unsolicited. (Later in this chapter, we'll cover the unfortunate exception to this rule when "patients" are hired to pose on listservs and rave about a doctor or facility.)

Involve your local doctor

You shouldn't have to be secretive about seeking second or third opinions. When you or a loved one is facing a serious medical issue, you have every right to gather as much information and assemble the best team to help you deal with your condition. When you find the top one or two physician experts in your disease category, you should certainly discuss your findings with your local doctor. He or she might want to speak directly to the expert and they may invite you to join in. With the advent of integrated medicine (the patient-centered practice of treating the whole person by marrying modern medical science with ancient healing systems), you might choose to have an acupuncturist, a naturopath, a massage therapist or a chiropractor on your team. It's important that you get these providers talking to one another and on the same page. After you have identified additional health resources to help you, it is important to remember that the more coordinated your care, the better. Don't stress out about whether you can make a big trip to see the top expert. Many will provide telephone or written consultations and record interviews. Even if you never see the expert in person, he or she might offer important guidance to your local doctor and other team members that will dictate the direction of your case. I often see the expert in that case as the architect of your care and the local doctor as the general contractor. As you would expect, it's important for the architect to explain his blueprint to the contractor and answer questions so you get the best possible result. Just as in a building project, things change along the way. The contractor goes back to the architect for further guidance. Same thing with changes or updates to your treatment plan.

Don't automatically reject local advice

Be careful not to discount your local physician's recommendations or referrals. If your general practitioner (GP) sends you to a nearby specialist, be open to the possibility that you may have been referred to the top expert in the field. Not all the cutting edge doctors are located across the country from you! Take the time to review the credentials of the nearby specialists to ensure that you're in the best hands.

Don't limit yourself geographically

As you look for the pearls, remember that the world is your oyster. The Internet puts global health care, along with all of its human resources, at your fingertips. Your expert may end up being on the other side of town, the country or even the world. If in-person consultations are unrealistic, you have the option of communicating and forwarding records electronically and putting your local doctor in touch with the expert(s). I have done that several times for myself, friends and family members. In such cases, the far-away physicians serve as powerful new consultants on your team. I have found that local doctors appreciate you making the connection – they learn from it – and it gives you much more confidence as you move ahead.

Do your insurance research

Unfortunately, health care is not free. If you are facing a serious illness and you have health insurance coverage, it's a good idea to find out in the beginning what your policy will cover. Also, if you want to pursue consultations with a national expert and/or travel out of your area for treatment, you should know whether your insurance will support your efforts. Some companies have regional restrictions; others have national networks. Start by contacting your agent or a customer service representative to learn your general options. If you do NOT have any health insurance in place (which is true for millions of Americans), you should learn more about what assistance programs in your community might be available to you. Contact the hospital to see if they offer support to uninsured patients. In addition, the U.S. Department of Health and Human Services has helpful information on its website at http://www.hhs.gov/faq/healthprograms/assistance/.

Reach out

When you feel confident you have pinpointed the one or two experts for your condition, don't be afraid to contact them via email or phone using the contact information posted on their websites. If your disease is the focus of their life's work, then that increases the chance that they will want to talk to you. Most of today's doctors are available via email, either directly or indirectly through an assistant. If you prefer a more immediate approach, pick up the phone. Don't expect to speak with them right away; you will likely need to go through office or facility staff. If so, be prepared to summarize your situation and be specific about your request. Do you want a phone consult or an in-person meeting? Do you have a short write-up you could email as a way of familiarizing the assistant with your case? Do you have your records summarized and up to date? If you want the expert to guide your care, you must be ready to send all relevant information. In addition, be prepared to take additional tests, even if it means repeating ones you've already taken. Most physicians prefer to work from their own set of labs and images that they have ordered directly.

Consider all phases

While you are probably focused on the treatment phase of your experience, remember to think beyond this chapter to the ones that follow so that you can bolster yourself with the experts in those areas as well. For example, over the course of her patienthood, a breast cancer patient may ultimately deal with specialists in radiology, pathology, surgery, radiation oncology, medical oncology (chemotherapy), reconstruction and rehabilitation. She should feel confident that she has the finest team assembled on her behalf during all phases of her illness and recovery. Medicine does not need to be a one-stop shop, so feel free to browse. There are advantages to staying in one place but only if the clinical care is superb. The recent trend toward multi-disciplinary care serves the careful doctor shopper well.

THE FINEST FACILITIES

At 66 years old, Barry Anderson was surprised to hear that the two main arteries in his heart were 95 percent blocked. He had no pain or shortness of breath, so he was shocked after a routine exam when his doctors told him he needed bypass surgery – maybe even a quadruple bypass to clear all arteries, including those that were less blocked but still a concern.

"I did some research in this and (found that) while this operation is fairly routine, they crack your chest open and harvest a vein out of your leg," Barry says. "Everybody I spoke to said that those two things brought the worst pain and aggravation down the line. Also, they wire your chest closed. And in 2008 the idea of somebody wiring my chest closed just sort of made me feel like, 'Where are our technical advances?'"

So Barry hit the Web looking for alternatives. He learned about a minimally invasive procedure that doctors performed at a university hospital in his own state. "I found on the Internet that this was (endoscopic surgery) done by a robot, with no cracking of the chest, no harvesting of a vein," Barry reports. "Moreover, they used a thoracic artery, which has a longer 'shelf life' than a vein that's operating as an artery. Recovery time is minimal compared to the standard chest-cracking, vein-harvesting procedure."

For Barry, a veteran, going to a facility where he felt well cared for on both the physical and emotional levels was a huge factor. "I spent some time in hospitals when I came back from Vietnam, and I am hospital-phobic," he admits. "I was scared. But when I came out of the intensive care unit after my heart procedure, people were just extraordinary. It was a wonderful experience."

Barry Anderson took the initiative to research his options. He discovered a facility *in his own state* that offered a better procedural alternative than the one his first team of doctors had recommended. His story is a great example of how to use the Internet to seek out where to get the best treatment. In his case, this led him to a top-of-the-line team as well (the "who").

A few tips on searching for suitable facilities:

Match the "who" with the "where"

After you identify the top docs in your category, match them with the facilities where they practice or perform procedures. This will be your starting list of hospitals on which to conduct research. This may end up being the only list you need, provided that the physicians you choose are affiliated with facilities you find acceptable. If, on the other hand, your research shows that your favorite doctor's facility is questionable, then continue down your list of doctors until you find one whose hospital is also rated highly. The goal is to find an excellent doctor who is connected to an excellent facility.

Read the rankings

National hospital rankings are useful when it comes to evaluating facilities, and the best of these comes from *U.S. News and World Report* (posted at http://health. usnews.com/sections/health/best-hospitals). The hospitals included in these lists, organized by disease category, tend to be affiliated with where the important research is taking place. They are ranked according to their success rates with difficult cases, rather than run-of-the-mill procedures.

Study websites

Carefully review the website of each of the facilities you're considering to get a sense of their clinical quality and messaging strategy. Is the site patient-friendly? Does it include contact information for medical staff and administrators who can help you if you have a question or concern? Are doctors' credentials listed in full? Does it appear welcoming to online and in-person visitors? Does it mention the age of the building(s) and equipment? Does it appear to reflect a realistic picture of the place or does it appear more like a commercial? Look at the site with a critical consumer's eye to help distinguish real substance from mere marketing fluff.

Review advertising

If your research turns up advertising content for a facility you're studying, look to see if the messages focus on the hospital's equipment more than anything else. While you want a place to have state-of-the-art devices, it must also have the experienced personnel on-site who are best equipped to use such tools.

Study the quality ratings

Quality ratings are often tied to infection rates. This means that if you identify a possible hospital but learn that its patients suffer from higher-than-average infections during their stays, you should cross that place off of your list and move on. Even if the world's greatest surgeon operates there, he or she is only as effective as the surgical team's weakest link. You do not want that weak link to be in charge of infection control! To review related statistics, go to the websites of the Centers for Disease Control and Prevention (www.cdc.gov), the

American Hospital Association (www.aha.org) or your state's health department.

Find a place where your case is common

Ideally, you should go to a hospital where yours is not the first case of its kind to be seen. You want your team to be experienced in how to address the nuances of your condition. This is one time when you do not want to be unique.

Look for multidisciplinary teams

With the advent of integrated care, patients benefit enormously from multidisciplinary teams. Unfortunately, not all hospitals have adjusted to this trend yet, so make sure you choose one that has. In this model, doctors from all points along a patient's care continuum meet regularly to discuss the big- and small-picture components of the case. For example, the team for a woman with breast cancer would include a surgeon, a medical oncologist, a radiologist, a radiation oncologist and a pathologist. Together, they decide on the best course of action from all medical angles.

Don't be sentimental

Just because you had a baby at a certain hospital or your Uncle Ernie had his gall bladder removed there does not necessarily mean that you should go there for lung cancer treatment. A facility can be great in one department and weaker in another, so be sure you focus only on what you're dealing with right now. There is no value in loyalty or allegiance when it comes to saving your life.

A NOTE ON CLINICAL TRIALS

Clinical trials test drugs and procedures in carefully controlled and monitored conditions in order to evaluate their effectiveness. Patients sign up voluntarily to serve as research subjects in these experimental approaches. Every FDA-approved pharmaceutical has been subject to a clinical trial. As an empowered patient, you may want to research the types of clinical trials available now or in the near future in your disease category.

In some cases – mine included – you might choose a particular doctor or facility based on where a certain clinical trial is being conducted. Some clinical trials are only run through a single medical center, so if you want to partici-pate in that trial, you must affiliate with that facility in some capacity.

If you want to seek out a specific doctor who also hap-pens to be a researcher at an academic medical center, you may have better luck if you present yourself as a potential enrollee in a trial. Nobody will ever force you to sign up, but researchers are always on the lookout for research subjects. If you come to them with an interesting clinical case, you might get more attention because the doctors are focused on advancing their research.

There are some risks of participating in a clinical trial. You will be experimenting, along with the research scien-tists, with a new, unproven treatment approach. If it is not effective for you, you might end up losing valuable time that might have otherwise been spent on traditional therapies whose success rates are better documented.

There are also some significant potential upsides. If you have full faith in the supervising researchers and feel confident that they have matched you to the right trial, you may end up as one of the first patients to benefit from the latest science related to your condition. That's what happened to me and I think I am alive and healthy today because I took that "plunge."

There is no right or wrong answer when you ask the question, "Do I want to participate in a trial?" It is an extremely personal decision and you should base your choice on a combination of professional advice (what your doctors recommend), education (what you've learned as an empowered patient) and instinct (what your gut tells you).

In my case, I tend to be a risk taker and an early adopter of technology. So that set me up to be willing to try something experimental and new. But when you go into a cancer clinical trial as I did, we're talking about very powerful medicine that, if used incorrectly, could kill. All the papers patients sign (and I signed many) warn of the experimental nature of the trial and that not all answers are known.

The same resource that connected me with the right doctors – my online community of patients – connected me with the trial. Not surprisingly, several of these CLL patients were already in the same clinical trial that was being suggested to me. So I did the obvious: I put a message out to the community indicating I was thinking of enrolling in the trial. I asked whether anyone had personal experience with it and whether they would be willing to speak with me by phone. Before long I was talking to a roofing contractor from Texas. He was a couple of months into the trial. Later, I spoke with a woman back east. Those conversations, combined with the trust I had in my researcher-physician and my natural bent to try something new, led me to sign on the dotted line.

It's important to remember that the standard treatments in my illness were not great, so the promise of the trial was that the result would be better. Now, all these years later, it has been validated around the world that I made the right choice.

Most trials are posted by disease at www.clinicaltrials. gov, a service of the U.S. National Institutes of Health.

THE PATH-FINDING PATIENTS

Dave deBronkart did not set out to be a noted patient advocate – vocal via his blog about being an engaged, empowered patient. But neither did he expect to be diagnosed in his late 50s with stage IV grade 4 renal cell carcinoma (kidney cancer at a dangerously advanced point). When cancer entered his world, so too did Dave's involvement in the "e-patient" movement, also known as "participatory medicine."

Dave's physician guided him toward online patient communities from the very beginning. "I had the good fortune of being steered in the right place by my doctor, who had been promoting patient empowerment since before I met him," Dave reports. "He 'prescribed' the Association of Cancer Online Resources, handing me a prescription slip that had ACOR's information on it."

A long-time virtual community member ("I started playing with CompuServe way back in 1989, years before the Web was born," he says), Dave was familiar with the idea of interacting with others electronically. So he logged onto ACOR's kidney cancer patient community and "lurked" for a few days, observing how members gave direct advice about where fellow patients should seek treatment and from what doctors. It struck him how honest the patients were with one another. "In the patient community, I found straight answers from people in my exact situation," he recalls.

Insider's Tip:

Insist on a team of health care professionals who support your desire to be an empowered patient.

Supported by his doctor and bolstered by the wisdom of his fellow patients, Dave pursued a clinical trial of an aggressive form of treatment for his condition. "Here I am years later and I'm completely well; back to normal," he says. "It's as if nothing had ever happened; as if I bungee-jumped off the cliff of life and bounced back up."

Dave began a blog ("The New Life of Patient Dave") to journal about what he refers to as his "free replay on the game of life." A few months later, he discovered the e-patient participatory medicine community and realized it perfectly matched his convictions about patient involvement. So he renamed his blog "The New Life of e-Patient Dave" (posted at patientdave.blogspot.com) and has since created a website at www.ePatientDave.com.

He even helped formalize the e-patient think tank into the Society for Participatory Medicine (at www.participatorymedicine.org), for which he serves as co-chair and which publishes the *Journal of Participatory Medicine*. (I am honored to also sit on the editorial board for the *Journal*.)

If, at some point down the road, "e-Patient Dave" deBronkart finds himself facing another big diagnosis, he knows exactly how he'll respond. "I'll drop everything and find the world's best patient community for that condition. It's the first thing to do."

Here are some ways you can navigate the online patient world to help your own situation:

Find the advocacy groups

Patient advocacy groups affiliated with national associations are a great place to start when you want to connect with others in your situation. (Think American Heart Association, American Cancer Society, etc.) Nearly all bona-fide groups devoted to research, education and awareness of a given disease have patient advocacy branches. And all the information contained on an advocacy group website must be approved and verified by its medical advisory board, so chances are good that the information will be accurate and helpful. However, the "official" content doesn't always change as quickly as the patient buzz does, so be sure to look for pages where patients and caregivers are allowed to post their own content. You will find a wealth of information from savvy, experienced, empathetic patients who know firsthand how eager you are to resolve your health crisis. Patients represent the most motivated segment of the health care population, so others who have walked in your shoes understand your desire for the best doctors, the most effective treatment and the most promising prognosis.

Identify the independent patient leaders

Whether or not they are tied to a national or regional organization, some individual patients stand out as leaders. They speak at conferences, maintain blogs about patient empowerment, facilitate online support groups and sometimes form their own advocacy groups. (The Association of Cancer Online Resources is a great example.) Chances are, if you can find them through online searches, they are available to you and other patients in your disease category. Often they are so well connected that they can put you in touch with staff at doctors' offices, helping you cut through the bureaucracy and get right to schedulers and/or physician assistants. (GrannyBarb Lackritz gave me the number of Dr. Keating's personal secretary and told me to use her name when I first called Houston.)

Be selective

Don't let your fear and worry overpower healthy skepticism when you come across patient mentors who seem too good to be true. There are many enthusiastic patients online who are extremely vocal and persuasive because they want to engage other patients. But before you listen to their advice and fly across the country to see their doctor, make sure that their expertise applies specifically to your situation. They may be passionate and prolific on the Web, but if their knowledge does not extend into your unique area then you should find someone else who is better equipped to support YOU. (I had an online CLL buddy urge me to get a bone marrow transplant, going so far as to warn me that if I didn't, I would likely die. I opted not to, and here I am alive and well.) The same rule applies to seeking patient support as seeking physician support: There is no value in loyalty or allegiance when it comes to saving your life.

Watch for plants

One reality of medical marketing is that some companies hire consumers who have done well with their products (drugs, devices, surgical procedures, etc.) to join patient groups and serve as hidden spokespersons. Granted, there is nothing wrong with shouting from the mountaintop about the success of medical victories. That's what patient advocacy is all about. But as someone searching for advice and support, you should be wary of the input of hired guns. When someone engages you in a more detailed online conversation and begins to point you in a specific direction, simply ask, "Are you a paid spokesperson?" If the answer is "yes," you have the option of thanking them and moving on because you then know they have an agenda. Accepting money to tout the virtues of a course of treatment doesn't make that treatment bad; it simply means that you should factor the endorsement deal into your overall decision-making process. The vast majority of online patients are motivated by nothing more than health and longevity and do what they do in order to support global patient empowerment. However, be aware of those few who are paid to point others toward their sponsors. Patient advocacy should be completely transparent.

THE NOT-SO-DELICATE BALANCE

The key to patient empowerment is complementing your doctor's professional insights with your own fierce desire to steer yourself back to health. Nobody will be as committed to your treatment and recovery as you and your loved ones, nor will anyone devote as much time and emotional energy to the effort. Your health care team has numerous patients in their caseload, while you only have one. So it makes perfect sense for you to serve as one of the lead researchers on the job.

The more informed and involved you are, the more confident you will feel as you move through the process. As long as you respect professional boundaries and conduct your research responsibly, the physicians you encounter should respect and appreciate your interest in your condition. So get to work. You may discover life-changing treasure.

{ FIVE }

DISTINGUISHING FLUFF
FROM SUBSTANCE

See Past Promotional Health Care Content

IN MY EXPERIENCE

I spent the early years of my career as a television medical journalist before opening my own video production company, Schorr Communications, in 1984. Our team produced corporate communications programs for companies in the health care industry. Since the Internet was still years off, many of the videos we produced provided important patient education content that was otherwise only available in print. For the most part, these pieces were intended to be used for educational, non-promotional purposes only. (At that time, the Food and Drug Administration restricted direct-to-consumer advertising for pharmaceuticals and many medical devices, so the bulk of promotional messages were delivered directly to physicians.)

One day a professional acquaintance approached me with an idea for a project. He ran a successful medical marketing agency and was crafting a campaign for a client that manufactured an implantable device. His idea was to create an "educational" patient video that subtly promoted his client's product above all others but would be distributed to patients whose medical profile targeted them as potential users. The goal was to have patients approach their physicians and request the product by name, while simultaneously advertising the product directly to the clinical audience. It was an early example of how to combine dual "push-and-pull" marketing strategies, creating demand for a product by "pushing" it to doctors and compelling patients to "pull" the brand along.

In the days before direct-to-consumer advertising was allowed, these forms of communication helped to fill the information gap between the medical and patient communities. In a way, companies were performing a public service by helping to educate the end users of their products. Granted, most of the messages were slanted toward a specific brand. But these promotional/educational vehicles often offered the only materials patients could study on their own.

My point is this: Long before I became a patient or even an advocate for patient empowerment, I earned a living as a medical marketer. So I have seen first-hand how promotional messages wind their way into what appears to be non-promotional media. The experience of producing this so-called "educational" video (and others like it) felt disingenuous to me, but I recognized it for what it was: a marketing strategy put in place to build sales of a certain product.

My work in this area eventually led me to my next entrepreneurial adventure: creating HealthTalk Interactive, which began as a series of phone-in discussions where patients could ask questions of doctors about specific disease categories. This format (which evolved into webcasts as the Internet emerged) connected patients with medical experts in non-promotional, uncensored forums. Patients had the option of participating actively in real time or calling in later to hear previously taped programs. Because the shows were underwritten by unrestricted educational grants from medical and pharmaceutical companies, our sponsors had absolutely no control over the content. We now produce similar programs at Patient Power, where people tell their own stories about self-advocacy.

THE HEALTH CARE ENTERPRISE

The cold, hard truth is that health care is a multibillion dollar business. So as an empowered patient, you must remember to be an informed consumer. This doesn't mean that your doctor, your hospital, the designers of your medical devices or the makers of your prescribed medication are after nothing more than your money. Quite the opposite – it is in their best interest for you to do well. But you should remember that they face enormous financial pressures, and you are a customer as well as a patient.

As much as we want to think otherwise, there is no such thing as a commercial-free zone when it comes to medicine. Gaining a better understanding of the forces at work will help you cut through the clutter when you're searching for your own health care answers. The vast majority of medical professionals and facilities operate with integrity. The same is true of pharmaceutical companies. The point here is to remind you to think like a consumer as well as a patient and to make informed decisions.

SAVE THE BEST AND TOSS THE REST

The deeper you dive into your online research, the better you'll become at distinguishing promotional from educational content. You'll soon be able to spot:

- Editorial vs. advertising
- Fact vs. fiction
- Significance vs. hype

The Internet's greatest strength is also its greatest flaw: Anybody can post just about anything on the Web. That's fine if all you seek are goofy YouTube videos. But when you're looking for life-and-death information, you have to be more discerning. Online scams are everywhere and the price of Internet entry is low, so it's not terribly difficult to find somebody trying to sell you something. Just because a medically oriented website looks impressive does not mean it is backed by health care professionals. Scammers know that many people searching for health-related information are vulnerable – sometimes even desperate – and some take advantage of that reality. So do be vigilant. And don't be a victim.

Once again, information is the best defense. Strengthen your skills as a researcher and get to the heart of the matter as you review websites related to:

- Hospitals and clinics
- Pharmaceuticals
- Medical devices and procedures
- Health portals (such as WebMD)
- Search engines

HOSPITALS AND CLINICS

Most people understand what we mean when we use the word "hospital." Any operation that calls itself a hospital must be licensed as such by the state. But the term "clinic" is a bit trickier. Many hospitals have satellite clinics that serve neighborhoods or have specialty clinics for specific concerns (obesity, cardiology or hematology, for example). In those cases, clinics operate as mini-hospitals and carry the same credibility and quality as the facilities with which they are affiliated.

But clinics refer to a much broader range of entities. There are many people who call themselves health care professionals, wear white coats and operate "clinics" that are complete shams. And anybody who looks hard enough on the Internet can get a mail-order "degree" and call himself a doctor of some specialty or another. These are the kinds of businesses that often tout miracle claims and sudden cures, sometimes presenting patients testifying to the effectiveness of their techniques. They are also the operations that tend to be investigated by the Better Business Bureau.

The lesson here is simple: Stick to the bona fide facilities and watch out for the frauds.

When you review the websites and advertising claims of the hospitals you're researching, there are a few basic rules that will help you spot the fluff.

Read into capital equipment claims

If the hospital makes a big deal out of its expensive new equipment, sit up and take notice. (We're talking here about MRI machines, CT scanners and other big-ticket items that help set a hospital apart from its competition.) Yes, it's great to go to a facility that uses state-of-the-art technology. But your job as an empowered patient is to make sure it also has the personnel and the expertise to use the equipment properly. Make sure that the hospital has done more than simply write a big check to purchase the gear then advertised its new acquisition. It also needs to back up the investment by training doctors, nurses and technicians in how to use the equipment properly. This is where the art and science of medicine truly meet. So dig deeper into affiliated doctors' resumes to make sure they are fully trained and/or certified in how to use the capital equipment the hospital touts. Because without human expertise, machinery can be meaningless.

Check out procedure claims

If a hospital promotes its ability to perform a certain procedure, make sure that its doctors and technicians do offer that service. More importantly, find out if they perform that procedure *regularly*. Many facilities imply that they do particular surgeries frequently when they've only done them a handful of times. But once a procedure is performed a single time then that facility can legally state it has offered that service. As a patient, you want to have your surgery done at a hospital that frequently sees and treats patients just like you. You do not want to be a guinea pig when it comes to a complicated procedure. So come right out and ask the doctor, "How many of these exact procedures do you and this hospital perform annually?" You have the right to a direct and complete answer.

Find out about disease expertise

When you have the luxury of time to research your preferred hospital, it's nice to learn more about the level of experience a facility has in your given condition. Is it considered a "center of excellence" when it comes to your exact disease category? A hospital might be ranked extremely high when it comes to cancer care, for example, but not as high in the treatment of diabetes. Advocacy groups can help you identify the facilities in your area with the best track record for your condition. Simply cross-reference the advertising claims of the hospital with the recommendations from non-profit groups to determine the strength of the promotional messages.

Insist on a team approach

Many hospitals claim to use multidisciplinary teams, but make sure yours really does. Is there a facility-wide commitment to team care (where doctors from all points of the care continuum work together to support individual patients) or is it more of an advertising gimmick? If you're going in for surgery, is there a post-operative rehabilitation facility on site? If not, is the one down the road actually affiliated with the hospital? Does the surgical team interact directly with the medical oncologists (chemotherapy doctors) and radiation oncologists who administer care following surgery? If the hospital promotes its use of large equipment, does it have suitably trained personnel to provide pre- and post-care related to that procedure? Does the hospital maintain electronic medical records that are accessible to all members of your care team? If so, all data on your case (including test results, diagnostic images, etc.) will be available to every doctor involved in your treatment, which is a very good thing. The more data your team members can readily review, the better. If your hospital touts its team approach, just make sure they back it up with action.

Make sure patient testimonials are authentic

When patient profiles appear on hospital websites, you must think of this content as advertising. Even when happy patients' testimonials include their names and home towns (which usually means they are real people rather than invented characters), it is important to remember that their stories are sculpted by marketing professionals. It doesn't mean the patients didn't have positive experiences at that hospital. It just means they have been hand-picked as exceptional examples of the hospital's skills. Obviously the facility will showcase only the best examples of the best outcomes and offer only the briefest snapshots of those cases. Your job is to dig deeper. See if unbiased patient communities (such as advocacy groups) agree with the hospital's advertising claims regarding the patient experience. Also consider asking the hospital if you can speak directly with current and former patients so that you can engage in an unscripted conversation.

Investigate infection rate claims

Some hospitals post information about their infection rates on their websites. If they do, chances are that their rates are low (meaning the facility is kept clean enough to minimize secondary patient infections such as staph that are contracted on-site). You can easily double-check these claims by running the facility name through such websites as www.healthgrades.com. If the facility you're considering does not post its infection rates, you should research them yourself to make sure you're going to a place where infection control is a high priority. Often the hospital association in your state can provide information as well. You can also learn more about the broader topic of patient safety by visiting the website of Consumers Advancing Patient Safety (CAPS) at www.patientsafety.org.

PHARMACEUTICALS

Cathi Little[2] has worked behind the scenes in the pharmaceutical business for years, first as a scientist in research labs, later as a product director for oncology drugs and eventually as a marketing consultant helping drug companies with brand strategies and educational programs. By the time she was diagnosed with type 2 diabetes in 1995, she had firsthand knowledge of how drugs are marketed to patients.

"When you're looking at an ad or reading up on a drug, you have to get through the clutter of what's important for you to know," she advises. "You have to ask yourself what your goal is and what you're trying to accomplish alongside your physician. Then remember that the drug companies are allowed to tell you about how great their products are, but they're also required to tell you the pitfalls. You have to weigh your risk and benefits."

Cathi notes that there are many educational websites that have been developed by drug companies to help inform

---

2   Not her real name.

the general public about certain health conditions and the benefits of certain medications. She's even built a few of them. "Look at who's affiliated with the site, because it will help you determine its credibility," she suggests. "Does it have a medical center or an advocacy group attached to it, or is it run exclusively by a pharmaceutical company?" She also recommends looking at who is moderating chat sessions and webcasts. "Are they physicians? Professional educators? People with real credentials won't put their names on things with false or misleading information."

Insider's Tip:

Look for the <u>people</u> *and the* <u>money</u> *behind the messages.*

Patients everywhere can be as sophisticated as Cathi when it comes to turning to the Internet to learn more about medications. It's just a matter of knowing how to find what you need.

The American pharmaceutical industry generates sales in the hundreds of billions of dollars every year. Drugs help treat disease, maintain health and minimize discomfort. They are an extremely important component of modern medicine and help to save lives every day. However, patients do often have choices when it comes to medications. At the very least, we should look into the drugs our doctors recommend that we take.

Here are some things to remember in those searches:

Go first to the branded website

Virtually every pharmaceutical product has a promotional website. Most use the drug name as the Web address (www.drugname.com), and are considered "branded sites." Branded sites offer all the promotional content you need, as well as FDA-required details about the product. When your doctor writes a prescription for a particular medication, visit its branded site for a complete overview of that drug. Keep in mind that the site also serves as an advertisement for the brand. Content will be weighted toward where the drug fits into treatment protocols and where it provides the best solution. It will not examine the latest research in pharmaceutical treatments of your condition unless that brand features prominently in recent studies. Don't hesitate to ask your doctor why he or she chose this medication for you.

Go next to the unbranded websites

In addition to branded sites, the Internet also offers a nearly endless supply of what are called "unbranded sites" for pharmaceuticals. These have generic-sounding site names that refer to a condition rather than a product. (Think "breatheeasy.com" or "sleepbetter.org," for example.) While many of these sites are produced and maintained by legitimate advocacy groups, there are many others that are created by pharmaceutical companies to steer you toward their products as you research your condition. These sponsored sites may offer extremely helpful information to sufferers of certain conditions. But empowered patients will want to know when there's a hidden commercial agenda, to make sure the discussion is fair and complete. To find out if an unbranded site is underwritten by a branded drug company, simply look for any small copyright reference that mentions a drug company. Or visit the "About Us" section of the site to see if a drug manufacturer is listed as a top underwriter.

In other words, follow the money. Whenever a non-profit has a single funding source, chances are that it's a corporate enterprise. If it is,

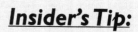

Insider's Tip:

Not all unbranded sites are promotional tools, but be aware that many are.

you have to decide whether the content is trustworthy.

Read the fine print

By law, prescribed pharmaceutical products must include prescribing information – the detailed disclosures commonly referred to as the "fine print." These facts appear in package inserts when the products are sold, in miniscule type alongside print advertising and in hastily read statements in TV and radio commercials. They are also posted on every branded drug website. If your doctor has prescribed a medication for you, you might be interested in reading the fine print to learn about the specific conditions for which it has received FDA approval, common side effects and patient warnings regarding potential complications. Granted, most of us would rather skip this and trust what our doctors have recommended. But the fine print may trigger a question for you, especially when it comes to how the medicine reacts with your body chemistry.

Don't worry about product loyalty

Once you begin taking a certain branded medication, you will most likely be added to that drug manufacturer's database. That means that you might begin receiving a steady flow of promotional content – via email and "snail mail" – that is aimed at keeping you loyal to that particular product. Staying on course with a prescribed medication is not a bad thing if the drug is working well for you. But if you begin to notice worrisome side effects, don't hesitate to alert your doctor. And don't hesitate to make a change in medication if that's what the doctor advises or supports. The reality is that many pharmaceutical products come with side effects, which is a small price to pay if the drug is saving or prolonging your life. But don't stay with a problematic medication simply because its manufacturer has targeted you as a customer and enticed you as a consumer. Keep in mind that in some illnesses, you can't change medicine the next day. Sometimes you have to be weaned from the old and even wait a bit before starting the new. But if the old medicine is either causing real problems or is not effective, it is wise to consider a different choice.

Medical devices and procedures

Before Amy Gray became a Seattle-based professional organizer and feng shui consultant, she worked with me at HealthTalk Interactive writing scripts, producing videos and making patient education materials readily accessible online. (In fact, this book was originally Amy's idea and she was instrumental in getting it off the ground. She is a talented writer and passionate about patient empowerment.) So when her husband's doctor determined that his congenital heart condition – mitral valve prolapse, otherwise known as a "leaky valve" – had gotten to the point where he needed surgery, she immediately got involved in the research.

"When my husband's cardiologist recommended surgery, he told us about a relatively new machine that performs the procedure robotically, which is much less invasive," she says. "The doctor told us we should fly to North Carolina because that's where the 'expert' in this procedure is based.

But I wanted to know if we could find someone a bit closer to the Pacific Northwest who was performing this same procedure."

So Amy sat down at her computer and searched the name of the machine. "It didn't take more than 30 seconds to find the site for the machine, which also listed all the doctors around the country who are trained to use it," she remembers. "I knew the site was going to be promotional, but we got what we needed from it, including copies of scientific papers and a video showing how the device is used."

Insider's Tip:

Some online research takes very little time. If you're confident you've found what you're looking for, don't add unnecessary time to your search.

She and her husband visited the two qualified physicians in Washington, located on opposite sides of the state. They asked the doctors how many of the surgeries they had done, how many papers they had written about it, and whether or not they actually performed the surgeries themselves. "They all have associates, and those surgeons are often the fill-ins,"

Amy explains. "We told each of these guys that we expected him to be the surgeon if we went with him."

Amy and her husband made their choice based on one of the surgeons' experience with the machine, combined with the relative convenience of his in-state hospital. "The rock star for this procedure is in North Carolina, but we found someone we trust and we don't have to travel 3000 miles," she says. They also felt confident in the quality of the hospital where the surgeon operated.

They followed the doctor's advice regarding the best device and procedure for Amy's husband's condition. They then found a qualified physician through a careful examination of the device's promotional website. Whatever initiates your device- or procedure-specific research, you'll want to be equally thorough.

Here are some things to keep in mind as you go:

Be aware of behind-the-scenes arrangements

If you are being steered toward a specific device or procedure as part of your treatment protocol, you owe it yourself to make sure there is a medical – rather than a financial – reason for your doctor(s) to recommend that approach. In recent years, there have been an unfortunate number of cases investigated and prosecuted by the federal government in which manufacturers have made payments to physicians in exchange for promoting their products to patients. While these illegal and unethical arrangements are rare, they do exist. Empowered patients must be on the lookout.

Reserve your right to a second opinion

When a physician insists on one product or procedure over all others, there is a remote chance that he or she has a financial interest in the transaction. If you suspect this, do what you would do with any serious medical recommendation: Seek a second opinion. Then consider seeking a third. The viability of the first doctor's recommendation will emerge with such added context.

Stick with what's been approved

Be especially wary of devices and treatment procedures that are promoted heavily on the Web but have not been mentioned by your doctor. Chances are these have not been reviewed or approved by the FDA, and the sponsoring companies are based somewhere beyond the reach of the U.S. government. Some such sites even post testimonials from phony clients who have been "healed" by the product or service. Others provide profiles of doctors whose certifications have been falsified. Just because people are called "doctor" or even have the letters M.D. after their names, it says nothing about whether they have the standing to give you information you can trust. Further, don't fall for the argument that they have a medical secret that the establishment doesn't want you to know about. Do you really believe if someone had a cure for cancer, heart disease or diabetes, it wouldn't make headlines around the world?

Remember the basics of empowerment

When in doubt about the legitimacy of a device or procedure, even if it's recommended by your physician, return to the empowered patient rule of thumb: Verify, verify, verify. Ask trusted physicians, seek counsel from your patient community, dig deeper into online claims.

Do what it takes to feel confident you're receiving the best care with the least promotional tie-in.

HEALTH PORTALS

Health portals are websites devoted to health care in general and offer patients a wide assortment of medical content. WebMD.com and EverydayHealth.com are two popular examples. Typical health portals are non-promotional and avoid pointing patients to particular physicians, hospitals or brands. They are supported by advertising dollars much like commercial television, radio and magazines. You wouldn't expect Nike to rig the outcome of the televised football game simply because it shows ads during the breaks, so you don't want a health portal's sponsors to skew its content.

When you visit a portal, you want to be sure its editorial discussions are just that – editorial. Are cancer-related articles weighted toward any one form of treatment? Are certain issues highlighted in a manner that appears unbalanced? Commercial support doesn't invalidate a portal's legitimacy; you just want to be sure it doesn't color it. There's nothing wrong with certain products getting mentioned in editorial content as long as there is a valid reason to include them.

SEARCH ENGINES

My colleague, Rachel Daniels[3], recalls that her rheumatoid arthritis (RA) diagnosis was confusing when she first received it in 2004. "I had been experiencing a string of weird things that sent me on little trips to the ER on weekends, but nobody could figure out what was going on," she remembers. "Finally I got diagnosed with RA, but it wasn't clear cut at first. They threw in a secondary diagnosis of Behçet's, which is also an autoimmune disease that can affect your joints and other soft tissue areas in the body. So I had these two diagnoses at the same time and they put me on heavy antibiotics before bringing in the specialists."

Rachel was working with me at HealthTalk Interactive at the time (she then joined me on the Patient Power team), so she was already very familiar with patient empowerment. "Being an informed patient, I did know it was something serious and I got right onto the Internet," she says. "Because

---

3 Not her real name.

I went so quickly from being a very vital person to being a slave to this disease, I went online to try and figure out what I had and what it meant."

By conducting her own searches into autoimmune diseases, Rachel sought to educate herself about her own condition because she felt she didn't yet have a doctor who was fully familiar with it. "I saw all these specialists, but each of them only knew about one piece of the pie. In our system, the GP is supposed to have the bigger picture, but it was clear to me that my doctor wasn't up to the challenge," she says.

Finally her rheumatologist found a medication that offered Rachel the best outcomes. And because she had conducted her own online searches to learn more about autoimmune diseases in general and her treatment options in particular, she felt confident that the recommendation was indeed best for her. "The drug the doctor put me on made the most sense to me," she reports.

Rachel continues to search for helpful information online as she lives her life with RA, but she is careful to wade through what she finds. "A lot of information is really lacking, just offering the basics without going deep down," she explains. "There's some good content out there about long-term effects on joints, stress management, foods to avoid and even tips on meditation. But I find that I have to take bits and pieces of all the sites because not one of them has the full perspective."

Insider's Tip:

When it comes to compiling the information that applies to you and your condition, pick and choose from multiple online sources.

Although she had years of experience as a health care education professional, Rachel's initiation-by-fire into her own patienthood led her straight to Internet search engines. She did what virtually every newly diagnosed person would do in the same situation. But she quickly learned how important it is to approach search engines with a discerning eye, since they can lead straight into the clutches of marketers.

(We'll take a more detailed look at search engines in Chapter Seven, but they are worthy of a brief mention here.)

Search engines are generally paid through advertising dollars. So if you conduct an online search, the top results you receive will be the sites that have paid to appear first. In addition, banner advertising appears alongside search results according to related content. Finally, because you connect to the Internet via a local server, the computer determines your region and sends only local advertising messages your way. This explains why you receive links to nearby hospitals when you enter a phrase such as "breast cancer surgery options."

One of the great things about advertising is that we can choose to ignore it. If during your search an ad pops up that intrigues you enough to click on it, do so. What you find might broaden your awareness of your condition or of local facilities where you can seek treatment. Just remember that you are responding to an ad that has targeted you by subject and location. Consider the content promotional.

THE MORE YOU KNOW

In recent years, members of the medical industry have become increasingly aware that they're not terribly popular with the public. Given the sky-high price of health care, the drug companies' impressive profit reports and the staggering percentage of the population who remain uninsured, there is a bull's-eye on the industry. Factor in the scrutiny of the government and the threat of tighter regulations, and health care business leaders – particularly pharmaceutical manufacturers – know that their livelihoods are on the line.

Patient advocates are cautiously optimistic about the trend toward self-policing among the for-profit branches of health care. Reputable companies are being increasingly careful, working more closely with regulators and offering greater transparency, all of which is good news for patients.

There is no such thing as too much information when it comes to patient empowerment. Do wade through as many websites as you can. Just remember to distinguish the biased from the unbiased so that you can weigh the information differently. You'll soon begin to recognize the sometimes heavy hand of medical marketers and be able to filter promotional messages more thoroughly. Being a more discriminating consumer will make you a far more powerful patient.

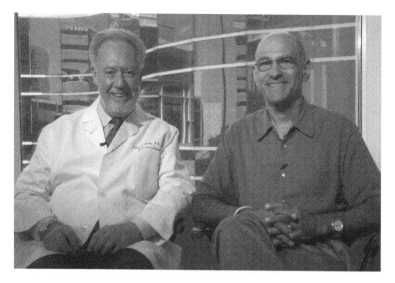

Andrew Schorr with leukemia expert Dr. Michael Keating

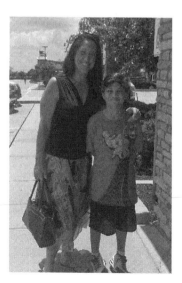

Beth Mays and Charlie (eosinophilic gastroenteritis)

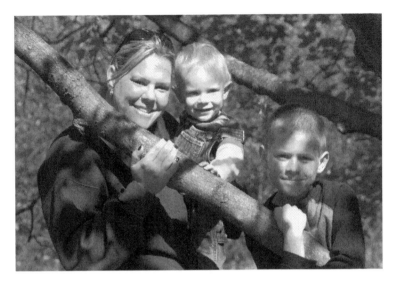

Jennifer Ambrose (appendiceal cancer) with her sons

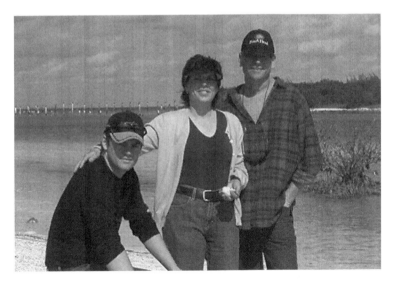

Patricia Beck (soft tissue sarcoma) with her husband
Rob and their son

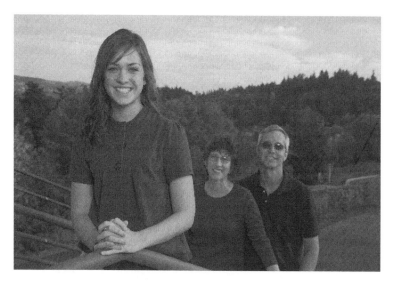

Katie Bunker (melanoma) with her parents

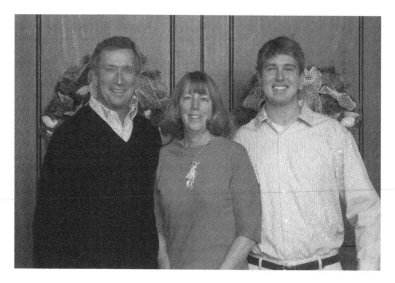

Gretchen Cover (leukemia) with her husband and son

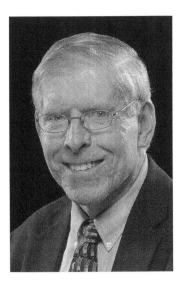

"E-Patient" Dave deBronkart (kidney cancer)
Roger Ramirez, Chariot Photo

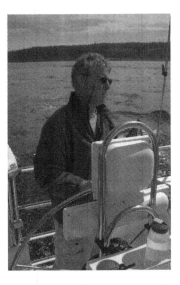

Ed Edwards (lung cancer)

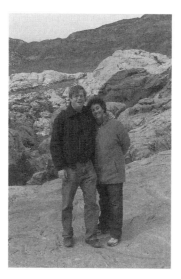

Amy Gray and her husband (mitral valve prolapse)

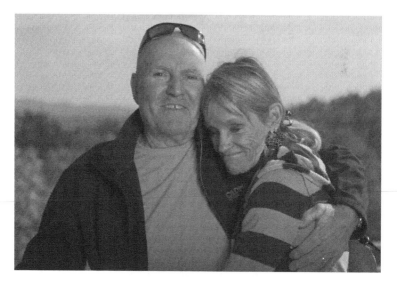

Mike McKelheer (prostate cancer) with his wife

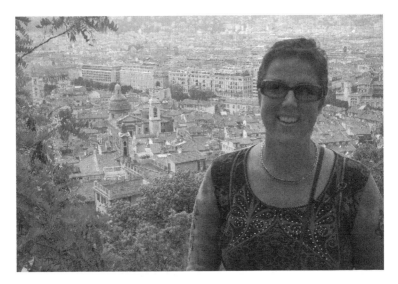

Jill Peterson (brain cancer)

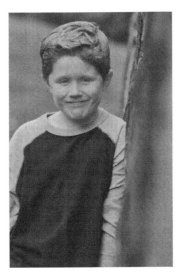

Cooper Reynolds (seizures)

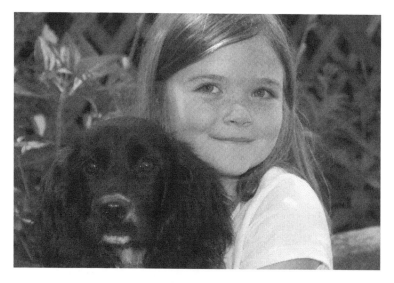

Molly Winiarski (phenylketonuria)

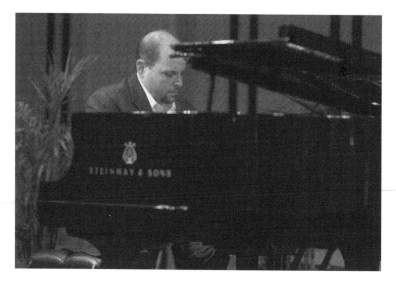

Matthew Zachary (brain cancer)

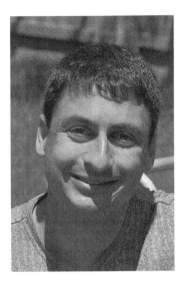

Josh Freedman (shoulder injury)

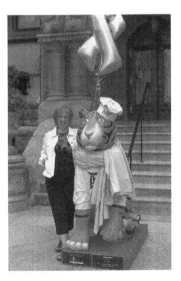

Valerie Fraser (inflammatory breast cancer)

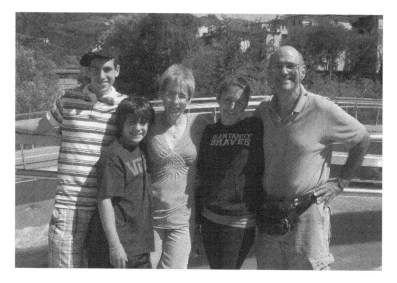

Schorr Family: Ari, Eitan, Esther, Ruthie and Andrew

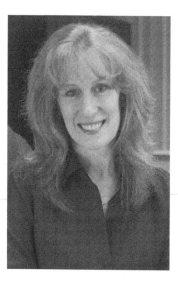

Lynne Matallana (fibromyalgia)

{ Six }

Reaching out to Family and Friends

Spread the Word and Get the Help

In my experience

When doctors first detected my leukemia in 1996, online mass communication tools available to consumers like me were limited primarily to email, and only some people had access to that. Esther and I spread the news of my diagnosis mostly via individual phone calls to family and close friends, which meant that we repeated the detailed report numerous times. It was exhausting and time-consuming.

By the time I went to Houston for treatment in 2000, the Internet was far more mature, allowing us to "blast" updates via email to multiple people at once. I had also spent the intervening four years producing informational radio shows and webcasts on CLL, among other disease categories, for HealthTalk Interactive (HTI). In these programs, I was extremely candid and detailed in how I reported my own condition and the nitty gritty of what it was like to live with CLL. People in my personal circle who were interested in my progress simply tuned in to the shows to learn how I was doing.

I've always felt strongly about speaking out about my health condition so others can learn from my experience, although I thoroughly respect and accept a person's preference not to do so. I choose to set privacy aside when it comes to my leukemia because I believe in the value of knowledge. If someone can benefit from my story, then the privacy trade-off is worth it to me. (The irony of a cancer diagnosis being handed to an established patient empowerment advocate is not lost on me.)

While I was in Houston receiving chemotherapy, I invited one of my HTI colleagues to interview me. So rather than acting as the journalist, I played the role of the patient answering questions and sharing my story. We conducted the interview over the phone as I was hooked to the IV on my second day of treatment, and I described the many facets of both the physical and emotional experience. The interview was posted immediately to the HTI website so anyone – my friends and family as well as the HTI audience – could tune in to hear my report. Since social networking tools did not exist yet, this rather unusual method of mass communication allowed us to spread the word on my status.

We were lucky enough to have a live-in au pair at the time, so our kids (aged 11, 7 and 3) were well cared for when we went to Houston. Whether we are facing a medical crisis or simply juggling the demands of family life, Esther and I have an incredible support system through family, friends, temple clergy, colleagues and professional counselors. We are never shy about calling on them when we need them!

CONNECT WITH YOUR VILLAGE

Someone dealing with a serious health concern today has a much more robust set of options when it comes to communicating with family and friends and letting people know what kind of help they can provide. These days most everyone uses email, has access to the Internet and carries a cell phone (many Internet-enabled). People are plugged in, which means they are easy to reach.

When managing your health suddenly becomes your full-time job, your "village" will be standing by waiting for reports and wanting to lend a hand. At the same time, the people who care about you want to respect your desire for privacy and your need to rest. Take advantage of the breadth, immediacy and utility of the Web to:

- **Provide updates** on your situation to concerned family, friends and colleagues.
- **Educate people** on your condition to help them better understand your situation.
- **Clarify the ways in which people can assist** you and your household.
- **Delegate** specific logistical tasks.
- **Communicate your preferences** with regard to visits, phone calls, etc.

- **Deal with critical situations** by distributing important information to help family members make important decisions.
- **Broadcast your research needs** to get outside input on treatment options.

Insider's Tip:

Using the Web as a communication medium allows you to distribute your news to a broad audience while establishing a slight privacy buffer zone around you. Multiple one-on-one conversations can be draining and become overly emotional.

PROVIDE UPDATES

Lindsay Wolfe[4] was only ten years old when she was diagnosed in 2004 with Crohn's disease, a serious disorder that causes inflammation of the digestive tract. Luckily for Lindsay, her doctors put her on a medication that eventually brought the Crohn's under control and now helps her manage her condition. But when the Crohn's first appeared, her parents relied heavily on mass email updates to distribute news to family and friends.

---

4   Not her real name.

"When she was first diagnosed, she was really sick," recalls Lindsay's dad. "We sent out lots of emails to let people know what was happening, what she was going through and the kind of support she needed. So many people came through by bringing meals for the family and gifts to her."

Lindsay's story, and her family's use of electronic communication, is typical during medical crisis these days. You want to keep people informed without having to repeat the details in numerous individual conversations. In addition, documenting the progress of treatment through a written journal can be as therapeutic as it is informative. (It also helps to track the chronology of the experience for both clinical and historical purposes.)

Consider these methods of online mass communication:

Email

Create a designated group of email addresses for those individuals to whom you want to send progress reports. Whenever you have an update to distribute, type that group name into the address field of the email message and all of those people should receive your post. When you want to add people to your list of recipients, add their email addresses to your established group.

Social networking sites

You can create a dedicated page on Facebook, MySpace or any social networking website that can serve as the headquarters for your news and information. You can post written updates, photos, videos and links to other websites that pertain to your situation. Social networking sites also allow visitors to post content and send greetings, providing an appealing interactive component. As with email, you can establish a dedicated group, including specific people via email to keep your page away from public view.

Twitter

If a health condition is in a stage where changes occur frequently and you want to provide regular, brief updates to large groups of people, Twitter (at www.twitter.com) offers an ideal medium. Each individual Twitter entry accommodates up to 140 characters, so it is great for quick, concise updates. ("Mom out of surgery. Doc says it went well. Please no calls to hospital today. She's likely here 2 days. I'll post again tomorrow at

9 a.m." This entire "tweet" contains only 138 characters.) Anyone who has elected to follow your Twitter posts will receive alerts when you upload a new one. Twitter is similar to text messaging in its brevity, but only requires that you send out a single message that automatically goes to anyone who has signed onto your stream. You also have the option of posting photos on Twitter.

Blogs

Whether you are the patient or the caregiver, you may consider maintaining a blog about your journey through your diagnosis and treatment. Blogs are easy to create and update and are available for little or no money. (Some examples of blog hosting services include www. blogger.com, www. TypePad.com, www.blogspot.com and www.webs.com, although there are numerous others.) There are no rules about how to structure your content; you can even think of it as more of a document of your personal journal than a public report. You can also incorporate images, video and links. If and when you are ready to share your blog entries with others, simply provide them with the Web address where your blog resides.

Video sharing sites

It may seem strange to incorporate video into your communications about an illness, but it can be an extremely useful tool. Consider the value of shooting just a minute or two of footage that shows a patient speaking directly into the camera and reporting on how she feels after an operation, then uploading that onto a Facebook page or a blog. More and more people are maintaining video blogs, choosing to speak rather than write their own words about what's going on. Videos can be shot with digital cameras, flip-style cameras or even with sophisticated cell phones and hand-held devices, and shared via such sites as YouTube, Vimeo and Google Video.

Educate people

Like Lindsay Wolfe, Katie Bunker was busy being a kid when doctors determined in 2003 that a persistently irritated bug bite on her arm was actually evidence of stage III melanoma, a potentially deadly form of skin cancer. As a 13-year-old, Katie was not thrilled about diving into treatments and hospital visits that took her away from the soccer pitch, the cross-country track, the dance studio and the seventh-grade classroom. She also hated the idea of people knowing about her situation.

As Katie recalled years later, "At first I was just so blown away by it I actually think I only told two of my friends — and I have a lot of friends! It was so difficult, even though I knew that they'd support me. Even at school, I actually hid it. I wore sweatshirts; I didn't want people to see my scar. I was always happy and friendly, but it made me self-conscious because I felt like I was really different from everybody else."

Eventually, however, Katie got to the point where she felt comfortable enough opening up about her cancer and discussing it with friends and classmates. Once she did, everything changed.

"Now I'm just spreading the word!" she says.

When asked what she would say to other teenagers who are diagnosed with cancer, she urges them to talk about it, let other people in and be open to their help: "Feel comfortable in your own skin. Don't be afraid to talk to people about it and express yourself. I wish I had spread the word more, but I kind of kept it closeted. It was definitely emotional, and talking to people about it is definitely the easiest way to cope with it."

Katie is now a vocal member of the melanoma patient community, speaking publicly about her experiences to educate others. "I like tell-

Insider's Tip:

Re-focusing your attention on educating others is one of the most effective ways of converting fear into empowerment. The more you learn, the more you can teach – and the more in control you can feel.

ing people about it now. I'm not shy about it whatsoever. My high school health teacher actually got really involved with sun exposure and teaching kids about being safe in the sun. I just love being part of this whole experience."

As Katie learned more about her own condition and became increasingly comfortable discussing it, she provided valuable information to the people around her. In many cases, patients have an opportunity to educate interested parties about the medical situation they're facing. When friends and family learn of your diagnosis, they will be eager to learn as much as they can about your disease. They may be able to offer more help to you if they are better informed.

As part of your communication plan, consider distributing links to informative websites you've found so that your support network can become as savvy as you are about your situation. You might even want to write up a brief summary, with or without website links, so that people can better understand your diagnosis. The more information your friends and family have about what's going on with you, the fewer questions you'll have to answer.

Send links to the specific pages that apply to your condition from the following sites so that people can begin to understand your clinical situation:

- www.PatientPower.info
- www.MayoClinic.com
- www.Medline.com
- www.WebMD.com
- www.EverydayHealth.com

CLARIFY HOW PEOPLE CAN HELP

Patricia Dunlap[5] of Northern California acknowledges the many "angels" in her life when she looks back on the grueling time when her daughter, Vanessa, was battling acute lymphoblastic leukemia, diagnosed in 2003 when she was just five. "Vanessa had wonderful doctors and nurses working on her at our local children's hospital, and I had food angels, cleaning crew angels and angels who helped keep an eye on Vanessa's big sister. We were just surrounded by people who wanted to help," Patricia recalls.

A cancer diagnosis is devastating to anyone, but it poses particular challenges within families where there are children living at home. When doctors discovered Vanessa's leukemia, Patricia's village went right to work to organize many ways to offer assistance. Patricia, a single mom, quickly learned about CaringBridge, a website that allowed her to post journal updates about Vanessa's status while also sounding the alarm about what she and her older daughter needed.

---

5   Not her real name.

"My work community immediately stepped in and helped me get organized," Patricia recalls. "They gathered email addresses from my computer and publicized the CaringBridge link so people could log on to see what was happening. One person from my office was my point of contact and she made sure that all of my professional and personal contacts knew how to get onto CaringBridge. It was a great way for people to find out when I needed food delivered to the house or when I needed coverage for Vanessa's sister."

CaringBridge allowed Patricia to marshal the efforts of loved ones, document her family's journey and do a bit of venting. "Another parent I met at the children's hospital led us to CaringBridge," Patricia recalls. "She told me I'd feel overwhelmed by the outpouring of support, but that I'd get tired of giving the same report. Once I got started with it, it became a huge part of my routine and I sometimes used it to get things off my chest. I was often up all night in the hospital anyway, so I made use of the time by posting updates and photos. It was my journal of that time, and it was a great tool."

Insider's Tip:

Maintaining on online journal can be as much about venting as it is about reporting.

Vanessa's treatment was successful and the family has shifted its attention away from cancer. "We kept the CaringBridge posts going for a couple of milestone markers, but life moved on," Patricia says. "I have so many other things in the moment that matter now, but it was great therapy at the time."

Patricia's co-workers made terrific use of an online tool to support a family who suddenly needed huge amounts of assistance. By designating an individual in charge of communicating when Patricia couldn't do that herself, she kept the lines of communication open and identified exactly how people could offer the help she needed.

DELEGATE TASKS

This is one of those times when you will need to become comfortable with the idea of asking for help. You will not have time to sweat the small stuff (taking the cans to the curb on garbage day or making sure the water bill is paid) as you tackle the big stuff (your health or that of a loved one). And there is a potential role for everybody, at every age and stage, when it comes to supporting someone they care about.

I recognize that you don't have to use the Web to delegate but my view is that it can simplify and speed up the process. No matter what, your job is to get well and to follow the orders of the doctors you trust. For now, leave the more mundane details to other members of your tribe.

The best thing to do for yourself and all of those people who are clamoring to help is to assemble your central team and appoint one person – to continue the sports metaphor – to be the quarterback. If you're not a football fan, think of this individual as your chief deputy, your right hand, your trusted advisor. In the following section, we'll use the title "point person."

Note: These tips are equally valuable whether you delegate using online tools or you choose to seek help and support the "old fashioned" offline way.

Here's how it works:

Name your point person

This person will act as the primary liaison between you and the rest of the family, friends, neighbors, co-workers, congregants and passersby who are eager to do something to ease your burden but don't quite know how to be the most help. Think of someone you trust implicitly but who is one step away from the immediate health crisis. (For example, a spouse may not be the best choice, because he or she will face the same time demands as you when it comes to juggling doctors' appointments and managing your household.) Your point person should be someone whom you wouldn't hesitate to ask for help of any kind.

Appoint a communications director

Although this job may be a component of your point person's duties, you should make sure somebody is in charge of getting the word out about what's going on with you. If you're comfortable doing so, you might share your email address book with this individual as a way of establishing the proper group of people to receive your news. Your communications director might choose to set up a website, a blog or a page on a social networking site. Depending on how you're feeling, you or your communications director can write updates and/or identify specific ways in which people can offer support. In some cases, when well-meaning folks ask, "What can I do to help?" and you're not up to responding directly, you can send them straight to your communications director.

Assign a food drive chairperson

The first thing people think to do in times of crisis is deliver food. By all means, accept the offers! It will relieve your burden and is the most natural way for others to nurture you. But first, put someone in charge of coordinating a meal schedule so your family doesn't receive 12 casseroles one day and none the next. Meal schedules can be incorporated into your online support site (there's a great tool at www.LotsaHelpingHands. com, along with other resources that help others help you) or done via email. Don't forget to remind your food coordinator of any dietary restrictions or food allergies.

Get help with your kids

If you have children at home and do not have family members nearby who can help care for them temporarily, you can ask a trusted friend to step into this very important role. Needless to say, you'll want to select someone who will take extra care to ensure that your kids maintain their routines as closely as possible during this chaotic time. The online communications tools that you select can include your children's obligations along with yours so that your helpers know about soccer practices, music lessons and homework due dates.

Put someone in charge of shuttle services

If your treatment schedule requires you to drive back and forth between home and appointments, you can allow members of your inner circle to serve as your chauffeur. You might not feel up to driving yourself and it's nice to have the company. Someone looking for a task can coordinate a roster of drivers once you know what your appointment schedule is.

Select a domestic issues director

This person can oversee all tasks related to your home until you're able to do so yourself. Managing house cleaning, collecting and paying bills, watering plants and arranging for a pet sitter are all jobs that can be performed or delegated by this individual.

Give jobs to the very young and the very old

Even a toddler can feel like a member of the village when asked to draw a picture to help you feel better, then watch as the scanned artwork is attached to an email message and sent straight to you. If an elderly relative is worried about you, ask if he or she would like to deliver a videotaped get-well greeting, which someone else can record and upload to your social networking page for your review. (All of these "assignments" can be made by your point person or communications director rather than you.)

COMMUNICATE YOUR PREFERENCES

You can also utilize any or all of the tools we've already mentioned to let people know your boundaries. The family and friends who are waiting in the wings are just as eager to respect your preferences as they are to jump in and help. So be honest and direct in stating what you need. Here are some examples of the kinds of information you can post via your online tools:

- Times of the day when you would like to receive phone calls
- Times of the day when you would like visitors
- Whether you would prefer greetings to be delivered via email or online posts as opposed to in-person visits
- When and where people can deliver food to your home or the hospital
- Dietary restrictions for you and/or members of your household
- The types of conversations you'd like to have (Do you need some comic relief or are you not in the mood for lighthearted banter? Do you want to discuss the clinical nature of your condition or would you prefer to talk about anything other than health? Do you want news from the community or would that make you feel isolated?)
- Special requests such as "no flowers" or "no young children visitors yet" or "no photos"

Insider's Tip:

This is not the time to worry about hurting people's feelings. Be clear about what will and won't work for you during this time. And don't be afraid to change your position as things progress. People will appreciate your honesty.

Deal with critical situations

If you're facing a critical or end-of-life situation where important decisions need to be made, you can use the Web as a bulletin board to post crucial information accessible by concerned parties.

If family members need to agree on next steps but are scattered throughout the country, one person can post key data to a dedicated Web page so that everyone can review the same unbiased, unfiltered facts and figures. This helps minimize confusion and inaccuracies during such an emotionally charged time. In addition, family members in different locations can conduct online chats to discuss the situation and determine next steps.

In some cases (such as when a person is still lucid but knows that he or she is terminal), the wishes of the patient can be documented ahead of time via a written document or a video segment, either of which can be posted to the dedicated online location. This way, when the time comes, there is little or no question as to the loved one's desires.

One might even choose to videotape a doctor's summation of the patient's condition so that the clinical perspective is available for review by all relatives, whatever their location. (Get permission from the doctor and/or the hospital prior to taping and posting such footage.)

BROADCAST YOUR RESEARCH NEEDS

Don't be shy about allowing members of your inner (and even outer) circle to supplement your research when it comes to your condition. It's possible somebody knows somebody who has been in your shoes or can offer insight into new treatment options available only in their region.

Use the Internet to cast a broad net, requesting input from all corners of your village. This is when networking can

Insider's Tip:

Tell a friend to tell a friend. Get the word out and deputize researchers in all parts of the country.

be a literal life-saver. People who care about you want to help, and this is one way to put their energy to a great use. Do send out the alarm for people's ideas. A loved one might live in an area where success rates are higher for the type of surgery you need or where there is a substantial number of specialists in your condition. You just might benefit from someone's familiarity with these regional differences. Or perhaps a co-worker of yours happens to know the head researcher looking for patients for a new clinical trial in your disease.

There are gaps in medical knowledge, and it's possible that your doctor isn't aware of a new breakthrough treatment that could help you. If that's the case, find out if someone else in your network can help you make that critical connection.

Just remember to employ your savvy skills as an empowered patient and filter what you hear so that it furthers your progress rather than clutters your mind.

Your village is your lifeline

Nobody should feel alone when facing a medical crisis. There are people near to you who are waiting to do whatever it takes to support you. Keep them informed so that they can nurture you through this difficult time. Be as open as you're comfortable being and get used to accepting help. You would do the same for them if the tables were turned.

Helpful steps to follow

Here is an example of an online path you might take to communicate to others what's going on and how they can help you:

1. Send an email to the people you want to inform about your situation. Explain what you know, including an exact description of your diagnosis with as much detail as you are comfortable revealing.

2. Include links to sites where people can become educated about what's going on. MayoClinic.com and WebMD.com are great places to start.

3. Provide a link to online discussions about your condition (such as those available at www.PatientPower.info) so your loved ones can learn more about the most recent discussions related to your disease category.

4. If you would rather avoid receiving direct replies, provide contact information for your primary point person.

5. Make it clear to people that if they want to help, they should coordinate their efforts through your point person.

6. If you have set up a dedicated website, blog or page on a social networking site, distribute that link so all comments, questions and words of encouragement will filter through there.

{ SEVEN }

DECIPHERING SEARCH ENGINES

The More You Know, the More You Find

IN MY EXPERIENCE

When our son, Eitan, suffered weeks of back pain and stiffness that his pediatrician predicted would go away but didn't, Esther and I decided to take him to a chiropractor. In my job, I meet and work with medical professionals from just about every specialty, but I was not personally familiar with any chiropractors in our area. So I did what any parent or patient would do in the same situation: I went to my computer, pointed my browser to a reputable search engine, and began a hunt for a local provider.

The search results included a number of chiropractors with offices nearby, so we chose one based on a cursory review of his website. The first visit involved little more than a quick overview of Eitan's discomfort and a brief physical examination. Then we were told we needed to return for a second visit to discuss the findings and next steps.

When Esther and I showed up for the follow-up, the chiropractor and his staff launched into what we soon realized was nothing more than a sales pitch. They spent very little time talking about Eitan. If we were to believe the detailed anecdotes they gave us over the course of two hours, this professional was capable of curing everything from asthma to Crohn's disease. He could also work his magic on Eitan, he assured us. All it would take was a two-year contract with his practice that he strongly encouraged us to sign that day. We made a bee line for the door, never came back, and have been happy to use the experience to warn others of this sort of shady practice.

We sought a short-term resolution to Eitan's achy back and instead were pushed toward a long-term relationship not based on any clear treatment plan. All because I found someone's name through a search engine and didn't take the time to research the provider's reputation.

Esther wisely pointed out that I, of all people, should have been more wary of such a blatant money grab from a seemingly valid medical professional. She was right; I should have been more diligent in checking his credentials. But it was an important example of how vulnerable we are when our judgment is clouded by worry for ourselves or a loved one. The mistake I made was assuming that the results of my online search included only websites and resources that were reliable, accurate and applicable to my son's specific situation. The search engine I used did its job to match my query. I just didn't do a good enough job evaluating the quality of the link I followed.

ONE WOMAN'S SEARCH PAYS OFF

Valerie Fraser describes herself as "very research driven" – a quality that she now believes saved her life.

Valerie noticed a slight swelling in one breast on New Year's Day in 2007 when she was 55 years old. Over the next several days, the tissue in the breast became thicker and felt hotter to the touch. Valerie went to her ob-gyn, who ordered images. Repeated mammograms were inconclusive, but a final ultrasound of the breast revealed two areas of concern. The doctor determined the problem to be an abscess, prescribed antibiotics and sent Valerie on her way.

Valerie wasn't satisfied, so she got busy serving as her own advocate, first pursuing the input of a local breast surgeon. "I felt there was something more ominous going on, so I called the hospital's breast center to see if I could get an appointment with the surgeon," Valerie recalls. "When they told me I would have to wait two or three months, I knew I had to get them to see the urgency of my situation." So Valerie asked the scheduler to show her images to the head of the clinic to determine whether or not the appointment could wait several months. "Five minutes later, I got a call back and I had an appointment scheduled for the next morning," Valerie reports.

Her instincts were correct: There *was* something much more serious going on. The breast surgeon ordered a biopsy, which eventually led to a diagnosis of inflammatory breast cancer (IBC), a rare and very aggressive condition that affects approximately two percent of breast cancer patients. Valerie's husband suspected IBC after conducting his own preliminary online research into her symptoms, so together they began looking more deeply into the condition even before the biopsy results came back.

"When we returned home from the initial appointment with the breast surgeon, I started immersing myself 100 percent into researching this cancer, using search engines to find everything I could about it, scouring PubMed[6] and medical journals for doctors who had studied it," Valerie recounts. "I figured that if this was going to be my diagnosis, I intended to become well informed and proactive in finding the best treatment. I searched for and found support groups, spoke with IBC survivors, read every study, visited every patient education website and consulted with specialists in my area. I learned that the experts were few and far between."

---

6   PubMed is a service of the U.S. National Library of Medicine that includes over 18 million citations from MEDLINE and other life science journals for biomedical articles back to 1948. It is located at www.ncbi.nlm.nih.gov/pubmed.

Valerie's research led her to a new drug shown to be effective in a clinical trial at a hospital thousands of miles away. So she took matters into her own hands and contacted the head of the study. "I hadn't even gotten my IBC diagnosis yet, but I described my symptoms, which had now progressed to include a rash, peau d'orange and nipple retraction. He asked me if I could get on a plane and come to his hospital the next day!"

Once she had her diagnosis, Valerie ended up traveling to the place where her condition was more fully understood and was treated by the research oncologist well-versed in IBC. She responded well to the treatment and currently shows no evidence of the cancer. "Going to the leading expert in IBC was instrumental in my outcome," she insists. "I urge other women in a similar situation to research and understand what they're dealing with. It's understandable to be blanketed with fear upon hearing or even suspecting you have cancer, but fear is paralyzing. You must move beyond your fear. Information is power. Without it, you can't help yourself."

Insider's Tip:

Arm yourself with information in order to make educated decisions when you need to.

THE SEARCH BEGINS

Valerie Fraser began her Web-based research the way most people in her situation would – via a search engine. Search engines help boil down the massive amount of available online information to manageable numbers of Web pages. They are invaluable, and we could hardly navigate the Internet without them. But they are only as good as the queries we submit to them. As users, we need to know how to ask the right questions in order to receive the highest quality results.

When you use search engines to research your health condition, it's important that you understand:

- How search engines work
- How search engines make money

- How to wade through multiple results to find what you need
- How to distinguish sponsored results from "natural" results
- How to make specific queries

An insider logs on

Josh Freedman considers himself fortunate never to have been in a situation where he had to hunt for information related to a serious medical condition. But following a shoulder injury, he wanted to educate himself about the short- and long-term effects of dislocation. So he turned to search engines – something he knows a lot about since he makes his living as a search engine optimization consultant based in Seattle. (Josh's firm, Web 1 Marketing Inc., has helped Patient Power become more visible to people searching online for disease-specific content.)

"I started by entering the words 'dislocated shoulder' to see what type of results came back," Josh recalls. "The first thing to do with any search is to see if the broad results are on topic and in the right vein for what you need. If not, you can drill down to get more specific."

For his own research, Josh then lengthened the string of words in the search field to include "rehab of dislocated shoulder." He continues, "At that point, I could begin to determine the quality of the information I was receiving. Some sites — like the local medical center and the Mayo Clinic's section on orthopedic rehab — attracted my attention more than others. They're recognizable names, and I am always more likely to click through to those, rather than to something less reputable like 'Joe's Sports Injury Clinic.'"

Josh's professional expertise gave him a slight advantage when he sought information for his own injury. But he, like all of us, began with a single query on a search engine. "There's just a tremendous amount of information out there on the Internet," he says. "You're going to find a wide range of quality and quantity on any condition, so a huge part of it is just knowing that you'll have to qualify anything you find. Search engines are great tools for finding information, but they have a very hard time evaluating it."

Insider's Tip:

Qualify search results with a few extra words to find quality information.

Be specific

The most helpful tool you can employ during an online search is specificity. The more detailed your query, the more targeted the results. So this is where we'll repeat the message of Chapter One: Do your best to define exactly what you're dealing with before you embark on your fact-finding mission. For example, instead of entering "seizures" into the search field, you'll get more of what you need if you enter "pediatric benign rolandic epilepsy" if that's the diagnosis your child has received.

With most search engines, you enter single words or phrases into the general search field and hit "enter" to begin the search. Some allow you to ask a question. In either case, you should be as specific as possible. Here are examples of specific and non-specific queries in both formats:

Non-specific (less effective): prostate cancer
Specific (more effective): prostate cancer, treatment, men over 50

Non-specific (less effective): what is prostate cancer?

Specific (more effective): what prostate cancer treatment options are available for men over 50?

Insider's Tip:

Start with simple descriptions and then get more detailed as you go.

THE MECHANICS OF SEARCH ENGINES

Since knowledge is power, understanding how search engines work might make you feel more in control as you conduct your research. Here's an overview of what happens when you initiate a search:

Search engines continuously send out electronic "spiders" to scan the Web and the content of sites, indexing what they find as they go. So when a specific phrase or series of words is entered into a search field, the search engine automatically pulls from its index and returns a list of sites whose content would match or get close to key words in the request. Since new websites are added to the Internet all the time, the indexes change frequently. Spiders also keep track of the sites that link to and from those pages to monitor related content. So when somebody enters a new search into a search engine, the system knows how to respond because of the work the spiders have already done.

With spiders working behind the scenes every hour of every day, they are able to deliver query results almost instantly. Best of all, the results are based on the latest collection of websites that have been spidered and indexed. (There is sometimes a brief delay between the time when spiders find a site, index its content and display the link in search results.)

Search engines look at a number of factors to rank search results, including:

1. Text on the site's page
2. The site's overall content
3. How other sites link to it
4. The URL for the page

Insider's Tip:

Check out www.RightHealth.com, a search engine for health conditions, which offers definitions, images, video, resources and patient forums.

A MULTI-ENGINE SYSTEM

When we think of search engines, we think of the biggies:

- Google
- Yahoo
- Bing

All of these services are backed by massive computing power, deliver quick results and offer easy navigation. They also operate in the background of most other online search functions that appear on third-party websites. There are more searching sites than there are search engines.

Still, you shouldn't limit yourself to any one of the most popular search engines because you can find very different results from one to the next. Think of how the Expedia travel website works: If you search Expedia for an itinerary in and out of Dallas, you won't see any flights on Southwest Airlines even though Love Field serves as the airline's headquarters. Southwest is absent among the search results NOT because it doesn't fly into Dallas, but because it doesn't affiliate with Expedia. The same rules apply to search engine results. Conduct simultaneous searches across all major engines to maximize your findings, since a site that ranks poorly on one search engine might show up prominently in another.

Insider's Tip:

Search multiple search engines to broaden the scope of your results.

SPONSORED RESULTS

Search engines, and the companies that build and run them, must make money to operate. How then do search engines make a profit?

It's all about the sponsored links, according to Josh Freedman. Organizations pay to have their products and services appear above and beside regular search results that pertain to their categories in order to get searchers to click through to their sites. It's known as a "cost-per-click" system.

Sponsored results are usually grouped at the top of the page where your results are displayed. In addition, there are often columns of sponsored links that run down one side of the results page. In most cases, the words "sponsor results" or "sponsored sites" also appear.

As Josh explains, "When a website's ad appears among the sponsored results in a search, it means that the advertiser has agreed to pay some amount of money each time someone clicks on that link. Also, the advertiser gets to specify where on their site the user is taken when they click on the ad."

Let's say that Acme Diabetes Products wants to make sure that its site appears at or near the top of the results any time a newly diagnosed diabetic conducts a search. Here are a few terms it might factor into its keyword advertising agreement with a search engine:

- Acme identifies a list of words and phrases (search queries) that pertain to its products and services.

- Whenever somebody in Acme's region enters those keywords, the Acme site will appear among the sponsored links at the top of the results page.

- Acme will pay a fixed fee (sometimes it's pennies, other times it's tens of dollars) whenever anybody clicks on their ad and is taken to the Acme site.

The sites that appear at the top of any group of sponsored links are the companies that have paid the most for the privilege. Remember that these may be perfectly reputable organizations that might offer you some of the answers you seek. However, just because they're listed at the top doesn't always mean they are right for you. Be a discerning customer.

Insider's Tip:

Don't reject sponsored links just because those companies have paid to play. But don't limit yourself to them either.

NATURAL RESULTS

The "natural search results" include all of the links that appear below and adjacent to the box of sponsored links. Once again, the scope of your results will depend on how specific you are in your query.

Broad initial searches, based on a word or two, will produce more results than you would ever want to wade through in your research. So add more detail to narrow your search, and your top search results will be more likely to apply to your situation. For example, when one enters the phrase "irritable bowel syndrome" into the Google search field, nearly 2.6 million natural search results are returned. When the query is narrowed to "irritable bowel syndrome, women, treatment, Milwaukee" then the results are narrowed to just over 35,000. While nobody wants to slog through 35,000 websites, this shows how quickly you can focus your efforts.

Your natural search results will include a mix of for-profit commercial sites, non-profit educational or advocacy sites and general health information sites. To gain a better understanding of your condition from multiple perspectives, you'll want to visit some from each of these categories.

Insider's Tip:

Review a mix of sites from your sponsored and natural search results.

SEARCH ENGINE OPTIMIZATION

Any savvy company with an online presence will do its best to be visible to customers and prospects. The best way to achieve that goal, explains Josh Freedman, is through search engine optimization. "Search engines try to identify the best resource for information related to each query they receive," he says. "Sites with lots of pertinent health information, as well as links from other sites, usually rank higher on natural search results because they're considered good resources for health-specific information."

The keys to search engine optimization, which helps bump sites higher on natural search result rankings, are:

- **Content**: Words and phrases repeated through-out the site's visible content that will match up with typical search queries.

- **Reputation:** Links to and from the site that connect it to other reputable, relatable sites.

CHECK LINK STRENGTH

Be smart about clicking through to sites that appear in your search results. Most of the links will lead you to perfectly trustworthy sites and, with luck, will yield helpful information. However, you might also run across sites operated by people whose intentions are less honorable. Identity theft and other forms of fraud are unfortunate realities of the Internet.

Protect yourself by following a few simple rules:

- If a site claims to be affiliated with a hospital or association, look carefully at the "Contact Us" page to see if that appears to be true.

- If you suspect a site is not trustworthy, check to see if the Web address is a slight misspelling of what you expected (e.g. "organdonor.com" vs. "organdoners.com").

- NEVER provide personal contact information via a website unless you have confirmed its legitimacy.
- NEVER provide credit card numbers or account information via a website unless you have confirmed its legitimacy.

Insider's Tip:

Most online information is free. Run away from anything that charges for info.

SPELLING AND ABBREVIATIONS

Search technology is getting more sophisticated by the day, and engines can actually correct your spelling for you if necessary. But it's best to spell words and phrases correctly in your query if you can. That way you can be sure to get the results that apply to your situation rather than to one that's spelled similarly but is actually quite different.

If you took notes at the doctor's office and are unsure whether or not you spelled things correctly, you can always check back with the doctor's staff to verify spelling before you sit down at the computer to conduct research.

Some conditions have long, complicated names and are more frequently referred to by acronyms. (PKU, AIDS and HINI are just a few examples.) If that's true for you, factor the acronym into your search to make sure you receive all applicable results.

Don't forget the library

There is no better resource for additional databases than your public library to supplement the work of electronic search engines. Either go in person to your local branch or log on from home. Many library systems now catalog immense amounts of archival documents and make them available to any card-carrying member. Library access is free, so take advantage of this wonderful old-fashioned research tool.

Follow the links

If you've ever bought anything on Amazon.com, you've also received follow-up recommendations for "books you might enjoy" based on the original purchase. You can create your own recommendation list for health care information based on your original search engine results.

Here's how to do that: Once you review your search results and click through to a site that proves helpful (and reputable), look for links to other sites embedded within the first one. Follow these electronic breadcrumbs. In most cases, sites with reciprocal links are designed to help you find the information you seek within your disease category. So rather than returning to your search results after you review each individual page, allow yourself to take a fork in that road until it stops being helpful. You can always return to your search results and resume your research from there.

Sometimes policy restrictions (such as at some medical centers and public health offices) prevent websites from linking to sites beyond their own boundaries. If you come to one of those contained sites, don't get discouraged. Just return to your original results and continue from there.

An ongoing process

Search engine technology is getting better and better, so we are more likely to find what we want right off the bat. As you become more familiar with your disease category – and more comfortable with your place in it – you will soon find yourself mastering "the art of the search." Your role as an empowered patient will strengthen with time and experience, so you will likely return to search engines many times to seek new information related to your situation. Each time you do, you'll have a better understanding of how to search and what to do with the results you find. Searching becomes a parallel track on your journey with your condition.

{ Eight }

Taking Information and Questions to Your Doctor

Prioritize, Summarize and Personalize Your Findings

In my experience

By the time I started seeing Dr. Keating, I was an active member of the online CLL patient community. This knowledgeable and empowered group of patients gave me invaluable advice on nearly every aspect of my life as a person with leukemia. So it was only logical that I turned to them for advice about how to approach appointments with my physician.

Prior to many of my visits to Dr. Keating's office, I posted questions to the listserv. Sometimes I confessed uncertainty about how best to phrase some treatment-related questions; other times I asked the group whether I should pursue particular subjects with the doctor. In each case, I received great feedback from fellow patients who generously shared their own experiences to clear the path for me. This online Q&A exchange helped me prepare for my meetings with Dr. Keating.

I later found out that Dr. Keating was an invisible member of the same listserv and monitored all of these online discussions among the CLL patients. So when I sat face-to-face with him, he greeted me with a sly smile since he already knew all of the questions I was about to ask him. This system was admittedly unconventional, but it helped to keep our appointments running very smoothly. We were both fully prepared in advance.

My patient community helped me zero in on the key topics to cover – plus things to set aside – when I did meet personally with my physician. I went into each meeting prepared with a prioritized list of questions, along with pertinent records and test results, so my doctor and I both got what we needed from our time together.

FACING REALITIES

Patients who conduct their own research will collect stacks of information and generate lists of questions to take to their doctors. This is an absolutely appropriate – and often vital – component of patient empowerment. But the realities of modern health care mean that in-person time between doctors and patients can be frustratingly brief. So it's not practical to expect a doctor to walk through all of a patient's research in a single office visit. The trick for an empowered patient is to learn how to boil down data and sum up questions to ensure that the most crucial points are covered in an appointment.

In this chapter, we'll talk about how to:

- Balance what you learn with what your doctor already knows.
- Respect the intense demands on your doctor's time.
- Edit and summarize your findings.
- Prioritize your questions to zero in on what's most important.

- Limit your communications to what applies to your immediate needs.
- Add members of your doctor's staff to your team.
- Supplement in-person visits with email communication when possible.
- Decide to go elsewhere if you are not being heard.

Insider's Tip:

Go into appointments with calm determination, not with emotional demands.

DOCTOR TO PATIENT TO DOCTOR

Elizabeth Morrison, M.D., M.S.Ed., has special insight into patient-doctor communications because she is a member of both groups. Dr. Morrison was a physician with a busy family practice when she was diagnosed with multiple sclerosis (MS) in 2001. Once she conquered her initial fears about her condition and learned how to manage her symptoms, she decided to make a significant career shift. She completed a fellowship in MS in order to open a clinical practice and conduct research focusing exclusively on the disease. Her dual roles help her stay on what she calls the "pro-patient-empowerment end of the spectrum."

"Patienthood has taught me how important it is to ask for what you need from your doctor," she says. "Sometimes patients feel they're imposing if they assert themselves, but it's okay to speak up."

Dr. Morrison considered herself to be a good listener even before she became a patient with a chronic disease. These days, though, she knows exactly what her patients are going through. "When you're really a 'true patient' you understand how hard it can be to explain vague or unusual symptoms because you've experienced that frustration of trying to convey those kinds of things to your own doctors."

Even before receiving her formal diagnosis, Dr. Morrison joined online MS support groups when she suspected she had the disease. She asked fellow patients for recommendations for an MS physician who would be aggressive with a diagnosis. "I knew I had MS, but the first few doctors I saw didn't believe me," she recalls. "When you know something's wrong, you want a doctor who will treat you even if you don't have a textbook case. I just wanted to be diagnosed and treated, so I found someone who was forward thinking."

Getting to the right doctor, stresses Dr. Morrison, is extremely important. Once you've located the person with the proper expertise, you should also be made to feel like a partner in your own care. "The right doctor won't be offended by your questions and your interest," she notes. "In my practice, we try to center care on the patient's needs. As a doctor, I wouldn't feel comfortable doing anything less."

Insider's Tip:

You may not fit into a tidy clinical box, since "textbook cases" are rare. Your case may fall into several disease categories, so continue to pursue treatment until something works, especially if you have been struggling with your health for some time. The knowledge of your condition may have expanded since your symptoms first appeared, so consider requesting a new round of exams and tests for a diagnosis that was initially rejected.

THE VALUE OF TIME

Time is a precious commodity. Patients want to make the most of it and physicians have to stretch it extremely thin. Doctors now make less money from insurance reimbursements and are asked to see more patients in a day than ever before. Typical appointment times have been pinched to as short as seven minutes, which leaves little time for discussion and none for in-depth review of complex or serious conditions.

If a patient pulls out a fat folder of resource documents and asks that the doctor review it on the spot (or even after the appointment), it places an unfair, unrealistic burden on the physician. The patient might feel slighted, but the doctor can't possibly devote that kind of time to each person who comes through the door. Also, if the professional deems the information irrelevant to the patient's case, then the patient needs to know when to defer to the physician's expertise.

When you have multiple questions and issues to present to your doctor, you must consider the limits being placed on his or her time. In turn, your doctor must take into account your desire to get involved in your own case. It's all about approaching appointments efficiently and with mutual respect.

Dr. Morrison recommends ending each appointment by asking the physician how you should get in touch if you have questions later: "It's always good to clarify in person while you're with your doctor because questions do come up after appointments end. Sometimes you can't talk to the doctor directly for follow-up, but it might be a question you can ask a nurse."

The idea is to leave knowing you can contact the office later with questions you did not have time to review during the appointment.

GETTING DOWN TO BUSINESS

As an empowered patient, you should treat every doctor's appointment like a business meeting. Set an agenda in advance, being careful to begin with the questions and concerns that are most important to you. Keeping your tone professional will help you stay focused and you'll be more likely to get what you want out of your appointment.

Prepare for each appointment just as you would for any business meeting:

- Identify the top agenda items for the appointment.
- Consider any additional resources that you need in order to deliver your key points.
- Bring any and all back-up data (test results, x-rays, etc.).
- Think through how you can support the doctor in her efforts to support you.
- Create a contact sheet with phone numbers and email addresses of all doctors who have been involved in your care.
- Summarize your past and current medication regimens.
- Print or write up abstracts of medical papers you think are pertinent.
- Assemble a list of Web addresses for any online resources you feel apply to your case.

- Provide a copy of all documents so that you and your doctor each have a set.

Insider's Tip:

Think of yourself as a professional patient. You will feel more in control and your doctor will take you more seriously.

A PRIMARY CARE PRIMER

Primary care physicians are generalists; they are the gate-keepers of your health care team. Unless you are on the short list of individuals who have signed up (and paid hand-somely) for "boutique medicine," you are on a long list of patients for whom your primary care physician provides care. The primary care physician's job is to evaluate your health by stepping back and taking the long view. If there are concerns that require specialized expertise, he or she will refer you to the appropriate specialists.

Note: If you have already received a serious diagnosis, you may already be working with a specialist. If so, your primary care doctor may not necessarily be a member of your daily health care team. If your primary care doctor is still your main point of contact when it comes to your health – which is sometimes true for patients with such chronic conditions as diabetes or depression – these next few paragraphs are for you.

When you get face-to-face time with your primary care physician, make sure that you focus on the questions and issues that are your highest priorities. If you are mostly concerned with the increasing severity of your asthma, then a discussion of your sore knee can wait. Along the same lines, if you are worried that you might be facing a serious but undiagnosed condition, be selective about what you discuss with your primary care physician so that you can focus on the key points.

Dr. Sarah Simpson, a clinical associate professor in internal medicine at the University of Washington Medical School and an internist with the UW Neighborhood Clinics, has been a primary care doctor since the mid-1980s. She has learned how to work with patients to focus on what's most important in each appointment.

"I'll have some patients who come in for a 20-minute visit and will want to do a full physical exam *and* manage their depression *and* their hypertension *and* their diabetes," she says. "I've learned to say that we can't do all of it today." In these situations, Dr. Simpson asks patients whether they would prefer the physical exam or the diabetes care appointment, and then she structures the appointment accordingly. As she explains, "It's better if we break things up over a few visits, and most people are understanding about that."

PARE DOWN YOUR QUESTIONS

I like to think of doing health-related Internet research as being like a first-year medical student. You start by gathering every single diagnosis that even remotely matches your symptoms. Naturally this leads you to some pretty horrible possibilities. Entering "headache" into a search field could yield diagnoses that range from innocent food allergies to life-threatening brain tumors. It would be a waste of your time and your doctor's time to storm into your appointment demanding an MRI because you've made the mistake of assuming the worst.

So simplify, simplify, simplify. Before each appointment, make a list of what you want to discuss. Then spend some time prioritizing your

Insider's Tip:

Becoming an empowered patient is very different than becoming a hypochondriac. Don't let your research make you paranoid about your health.

questions. You can even combine your top concerns with some of the findings of your online research.

When Dr. Simpson's patients attempt to self-diagnose, she recommends that they come in with their Internet diagnoses on the right side of a sheet of paper and a list of their symptoms on the left. "I'll listen with my medical ears and try to interpret the symptoms rather than jumping immediately to one of the Internet diagnoses," she says.

In addition, Dr. Simpson works with patients to identify which of the items on their lists are valid concerns and which are less worthy of their limited time. "I'll often ask them to give me the whole list, and then we negotiate together about what we get done today. That sort of helps us both get on the same page regarding what the expectations are for the visit," she explains. "I may decide to change the agenda if I find something really abnormal. So a person comes in and says, 'I want you to handle my fingernail fungus' and their blood pressure is 200/115. I'll tell them I really don't care about the fungus today; we're going to treat this blood pressure because, of course, that's what they would want me to do."

Insider's Tip:

Bring two copies of your list of questions and concerns so you and your doctor can each have one during and after the appointment.

START WITH YOUR CHIEF CONCERN

Before each appointment, try to think of the one thing that you want to accomplish. Is there a single question you really want answered? Do you need to come to a decision on one particular issue? Are you experiencing a new symptom that is bothering you more than anything else right now? Whatever your chief concern, it should garner the number one spot on the list that you take with you to your appointment.

Zero in on your main concern and kick-start your doctor-patient discussion with that topic. Even if you never move on to the next five items on your list, you'll cover the most pressing issue.

Most doctors will begin office visits by asking what you'd like to go over or if you have any specific areas of concern. This is your invitation to present your list. If "the big one" is at the top, then you've done the most important part of your homework.

If you find yourself with more than one issue that feels especially pressing and you run out of time, Dr. Morrison recommends simply asking for more. "It's your appointment. If you have questions, it's the doctor's job to answer them," she says. "If you don't get through them all, just say you want to schedule another time to come back and finish them later. The doctor might be really happy with this, especially if she's assuming that the patient wants to get through them all in one sitting. By setting up a second visit, it helps take pressure off of both of them."

GETTING PERSONAL AND KEEPING IT THAT WAY

You can review every Web-based reference there is and what you learn won't affect your outcome if the information doesn't apply to your unique situation. So when you bring things to your doctor – summaries of medical research papers, case studies of patients in your disease category, statistics on the success of one drug over another – you must be careful to personalize it to your specific case.

Personalized medicine (a hot health care topic) is all about determining what's relevant and significant to an individual patient rather than an entire patient population. Your responsibility when you serve as your own advocate, as we've discussed, is to be discerning when you research your condition. This is also true when it comes to presenting your physician with your findings. If it doesn't have to do with the exact thing you're dealing with, then it doesn't apply. So skip that information.

Insider's Tip:

Preparing for and meeting with your doctor is an opportunity to make things all about you!

Bring your complete file

Doctors and empowered patients agree: One of the best ways to keep appointments running smoothly is to bring all past and current records, test results and images (x-rays, ultrasounds, MRIs, etc.) that you have. Even if you think your doctor already has a copy of such records, bring them anyway. (We'll talk more about this in Chapter Nine.)

Doctors sometimes need these files well in advance of the in-person visit. Always check ahead to see if your physician would like to review your records prior to your appointment. Given how difficult it can be to make appointments with the sought-after experts, you want to take care of these details beforehand to make the most of your face-to-face meeting.

When my daughter, Ruth, was 10 years old, she was showing early signs of what we now know to be celiac disease (finally diagnosed when she was 16). I arranged to take her halfway across the country to see a noted pediatric specialist who would test her for various food allergies. It was difficult to get an appointment on this busy physician's schedule and seeing him required taking Ruth out of school for several days to make the trip. But we went to these extreme lengths because Esther and I believed in the value of having our child be seen by the best of the best.

When we got there, we learned that Ruth would not be able to take any of the scheduled tests because of another medication that she was taking at the time. I had multiple conversations with the doctor's staff but nobody had informed me of this restriction. I had asked lots of other questions about how to prepare Ruth's records but had failed to ask about how to prepare Ruth's body.

We did get useful information from this trip, but not as complete a picture as we would have liked. Six years later, with another world-famous specialist, Ruthie finally had the test she would have had as part of the total workup at age 10. Her test result at age 16 was negative. But wouldn't it have been great to know that long ago?

Ask your doctor (or a staff member in the doctor's office) these questions in advance of your appointment:

- Which of my test records do you want to review in advance?
- What tests do I need to repeat prior to my appointment with you?
- Are there testing facilities or labs where you would prefer that I go?
- What types of family history would you like me to summarize?
- What other documentation should I have with me at our appointment?
- Do I need to fast prior to the appointment?
- What do you need to know about my current medications and supplements?

The more organized you are before and during your visit, the less time the doctor has to spend interviewing you to uncover these particulars. So take care of functional details in advance. You'll spend more of your appointment time covering your questions and crafting your plan as a team.

Insider's Tip:

When visiting a doctor for the first time, make sure you know where you're going. Print out directions to the office, know the parking options and leave plenty of time to get there.

THE DOCTOR-PATIENT PARTNERSHIP

There are many advantages to getting organized for your doctor's visits. Most have to do with maximizing efficiency in order to make the best use of limited time. Another reason is to make sure you're working with the right partner in your care.

Sometimes there are differences of opinion between patients and doctors. Sometimes there are gaps in expertise on the part of physicians. You can determine whether or not your doctor is truly knowledgeable when it comes to your disease category by doing your own research and presenting your findings professionally and proficiently.

I do not mean to imply that patients without medical degrees can match the training and expertise of their physicians. I mean that every patient deserves to work in partnership with a doctor who demonstrates in-depth knowledge and a genuine respect for patient empowerment.

Don't be afraid to ask your physicians to be honest about the limits of their own knowledge so you can determine whether or not you want to seek other opinions. Keep looking, if necessary, until you can find a true partner in your case.

Remember that you always have the option of speaking directly to the pathologist (the physician who analyzes laboratory results and determines the presence or absence of disease) who has reviewed your case. Pathology reports include specific data that doctors often use to determine the course of treatment so feel free to request a meeting with the person who interpreted your tests and wrote up your report. He or she may be able to clarify your diagnosis and condition in a way that adds to what your doctor has already discussed with you.

Insider's Tip:

Be your own advocate, not your own medical expert. Balance what you learn with what the medical establishment knows.

E-COMMUNICATING WITH YOUR DOCTOR

An increasing number of patients express a desire to communicate with their doctors via email. Sounds easy enough, but this is a bit tricky. The Federal Health Insurance Portability and Accountability Act (HIPAA) requires that electronic protected health information, including email and medical records, be transmitted via secure systems. So doctors are limited in what they can say and discuss in email.

Secondly, there is some concern that if physicians begin communicating with patients via email, they will get bombarded with endless messages detailing harmless symptoms and non-specific complaints. If a doctor were to answer every email, he would have no time to see patients.

Thirdly, doctors are paid for office visits, not for time spent at a computer screen replying to email queries.

So the current system must change in order for patient-doctor email communication to become an everyday component of health care.

Despite all that, approximately one-third of doctors reportedly use email to connect with patients and the numbers are growing.[7] Some hospitals have initiated online programs that allow patients to email doctors and other health care professionals with specific questions or concerns. Dr. Simpson's clinic has such a program, which also helps patients inquire about – and even schedule – any necessary pre-appointment tests and check on test results online. "They can also communicate with us about new symptoms," she reports. "If it's something simple, we can make some recommendations on the secure server. If it's more complicated, then we say we really need to see them."

It's worth asking whether your doctor and/or hospital have any of these email systems in place. Growing demand from patients may help widen their use.

---

7   Chang, Alicia. "It's no LOL: Few US doctors answer e-mails from patients." 22 Apr. 2008. Associated Press.

Insider's Tip:

If you have access to your online records, chart any changes in your pap results, mammograms, PSA tests, cholesterol levels, blood pressure, etc. Perform your own comparative studies.

ADD YOUR DOCTOR'S STAFF TO YOUR TEAM

One of the best ways to get the most of your in-person appointment with your physician is to get to know and work with her staff. Nurses, schedulers and office managers are hugely important members of your health care team and can serve as crucial allies.

In advance of any big visit to the office, contact one of the nurses to make sure that you have all the records you'll need for the appointment. Are there any additional documents that you can help locate and deliver to the doctor's office?

Also, find out how much time has been blocked out for you and ask whether the nurse thinks the allotted time is sufficient to accomplish your goals for the meeting. If the answer is no, then respectfully request a longer appointment. It never hurts to ask; you have every right to do so.

In a hospital, there are social workers and patient liaisons who can also assist with some scheduling and logistical challenges in certain cases. If you don't get the answers you need from the first person who answers the phone at your doctor's office, keep going through the staff roster until you find someone who will help you. Be assertive, not aggressive; be persistent, not antagonistic.

Insider's Tip:

Medical professionals are busy, not untouchable. Seek out a helpful staff member at your doctor's office and don't stop looking until you find one.

CHOOSE COMPANIONS CAREFULLY

You put a lot of thought into *what* to take to your appointments. Do the same when it comes to deciding *whom* to take to your appointments.

Take someone with you who will support you, echo the tone you set and respect the fact that it's your meeting. Do not take someone who could derail the visit by being overly emotional or demanding. If possible, your companion should be well-informed on your condition and your current status. This person should not come equipped with a notebook of papers pulled from his or her own online research. Your helper should not do supplemental homework, as that will only complicate the conversation you need to have during that previous visit with your doctor.

Communicate very clearly how you would like your companion to help you. Explain whether you want him to listen or chime in. Tell him exactly what you need to support your efforts. If you don't feel the person can respect your wishes, then look elsewhere for an "assistant."

Sometimes the most valuable service a friend or relative can provide for you is to sit quietly and record the meeting, either in audio or video format. (Get permission first from the doctor.) You can then focus on interacting with your physician without worrying about missing important details.

Insider's Tip:

The right support person can enhance an appointment. The wrong one can steer the visit off-track.

REMEMBER YOUR OPTIONS

As a powerful patient, you want to do whatever it takes to maximize the success of every doctor visit. Being organized for your appointments is one of the most important things you can do. However, if you feel your physician and/ or your hospital is not meeting you at least halfway in that effort, then you always have the option of going elsewhere. Remember that option in case you need it.

When your health is at stake, few things are as pivotal as time. You and your health care team should be working together to use it wisely.

{ Nine }

Maintaining Your Records

Stay Organized as You Manage Your Files

In my experience

The Internet barely existed at the time of my diagnosis, so there were no online tools to help me with record-keeping. Beyond storing a lot of my own health information in my head (the most low-tech approach and one that I don't recommend!), the only data I consistently tracked during that initial phase were my white blood counts. I watched these numbers closely, as they offered the greatest insight into the progression of my leukemia.

However, in the time that elapsed between my 1996 diagnosis and my first round of treatment in August 2000,

I collected enough background information on my disease, my treatment options and my various facts and figures to fill a fat three-ring binder. (Esther was a huge help with this; she gathered and organized the entire section on my test results.) We took the binder to Houston, where we stuffed it with even more copies of documents related to my treatment. We continued to store records there as I received treatments in Houston and throughout my final rounds of treatments back home in Seattle (until February 2001).

Since then, I have gotten into the habit of filing any piece of paper with data related to my case. Whenever I take any kind of test, I ask for a copy of the results so I can add it to my file. My hard copy binder is the nerve center of my personal medical record because I created it before there was any such thing as an online alternative. Now that patients have the option of storing and accessing their records via the Web, I am slowly transitioning to this approach. If my medical situation changes and I need to track pharmaceuticals, diagnostic test results and/or treatment regimens, I will rely on the Internet to help me manage what can be an overwhelming amount of data.

A POWER SHIFT

Until recently, doctors monopolized power in the world of health care. They held all files, had sole access to all records and only released information to patients when they deemed it absolutely necessary. Today empowered patients may view and manage all their health care records. Numerous online tools make the process easy. Doctors and hospitals are even participating in programs that allow direct connectivity with patients.

This shift is extremely positive – I would even call it revolutionary. Electronic record-keeping systems are more accurate, easier to track and create a better mode of communication between patient and provider (as well as between provider and provider). It also puts more power in the hands of patients. Imagine how much time, money and emotional energy could be saved if every patient's files were stored in a reliable, accessible electronic form.

Being organized is always the first step to feeling more in control. Organizing one's medical records helps narrow the discussion, giving patients a better sense of where their health has been and where they want it to go. Visual learners can graph important numbers (blood counts, cholesterol levels, etc.) while research junkies can catalog reports that pertain to their health concern. You can track medication dosage patterns, store copies of diagnostic images and create a subject index of notes you take at doctor's appointments. There is virtually no limit to the ways in which you can digitize your records.

So now that you've done the hard work of researching and connecting online, the next logical step is to store your valuable collection of data in a secure central location. It's more than just a way to organize your health-related information; it's also a tool that your loved ones can use to support you, both on a daily basis and in the event of an emergency. I believe maintaining records online is one more form of preventive medicine.

Insider's Tip:

Organizing your data will save you time and make you feel empowered.

WHAT TO INCLUDE IN YOUR BINDER

Once you've become an information detective, you should have a logical system to file your findings and organize all data related to your case. Your binder – whether it's digital, actual or a little of both – can contain any or all of these items, categorized into sections:

- Diagnostic test results and related write-ups
- Lab reports and related write-ups
- Copies of images (x-rays, MRIs, scans, etc.)
- Trackable numbers (blood counts, cholesterol level, weight, blood pressure, etc.)
- Documents and Web pages pertaining to your research about your condition
- Contact info for all members of your health care team
- A list of your emergency contacts
- Your health insurance information
- Immunization records
- Videos of physicians speaking about your case and/ or about your health concern
- Videos of your procedures

- Links to applicable patient community discussions

- Personal diary or blog entries about how you are feeling emotionally

- Daily journal entries recording how you are feeling physically

- Medication logs with drug names, dosages, dispensing pharmacies and dates

- Official medication information (package inserts), including side effects and potential interactions

- Copies of powers of attorney and health care directives

Insider's Tip:

Your condition will change over time, so your files should do the same. Be flexible about adding new categories of information as the need arises.

MANAGING MULTIPLE RECORDS

Sara McKenzie[8] speaks for many of us when she describes her primary reasons for using online record-keeping systems

---

8   Not her real name.

rather than traditional hard-copy files. "I have a real knack for losing pieces of paper. It's almost a gift," she admits. So when she learned she could store and use medical records online, she took full advantage of the opportunity.

"When it comes to health-related paperwork, it's too difficult to discern the important pieces from the rest of it. Anything that's important in 'life management' should be stored online. That way, it's accessible and I can search and find it," she says.

Sara uses Google Health to maintain her own records as well as the files of her teenage daughter and her father, who is in his 80s. She even uses the system to help manage the records of a family friend who deals with multiple health concerns, including diabetes, heart disease and high cholesterol.

Since Sara and her daughter are both healthy, they use the service primarily for everyday record-keeping and learning more about their health rather than to manage complicated medications or diagnostic records. They find it helpful to track immunizations and other records needed for camps and school, along with things like monitoring weight and body mass index (BMI). As they make future transitions – if the family switches insurance, goes to a new doctor/specialist, or as her daughter moves from a pediatrician to a family practitioner – their files will remain in one central place and will continue to be accessible to them from anywhere.

"To me, it's not just about looking backward at historical records gathering dust. It's about using them to make the right health decisions today and in the future for our kids," Sara says. "As she gets older, my daughter will know her family health history as well as her own."

Sara's father is still healthy and active. But if a time comes when he needs care, Sara and her siblings know right where to find his medical history. "It was easy for me to set up his profile and give him and my siblings access to it," she says.

For her friend with the more complex medical profile, Sara helps log his over-the-counter supplements alongside his prescribed medications. If there were any danger of negative interactions, Google Health would flag it, another helpful benefit of online storage.

Sara points out another important benefit: "I now feel better prepared for emergencies, since having access to key family medical information helps me be a better emergency contact. I'm prepared to share potentially life-saving information if needed. My family also has access to *my* records so that my health-related wishes would be carried out in case of emergency. My phone is always with me and has emergency contact numbers. My emergency contacts have access to a signed and notarized copy of my advanced directive, also kept on Google Health. To me, this is just about being a good citizen."

A TRUSTWORTHY REPOSITORY

Like most parents, Christy Schulz has a lot to monitor when it comes to her family's medical records. Although she, her husband and their two school-aged kids are generally healthy, there are still numerous files to manage. Three major moves in the last ten years have complicated matters by spreading the family's records across various medical offices throughout the Midwest.

"I needed a better way to keep track of all of the files kept by all of the medical personnel we've been in contact with over the years," Christy says. "There was so much information spread out over so many different places; it seemed ridiculous to have to call each doctor's office any time we needed to gather medical history."

After doing a bit of research, Christy located a record-keeping system offered online by the Mayo Clinic. (The system is powered by Microsoft HealthVault). "It was one repository where I could hold all that information that we'd encountered over the years," she explains. "I don't even use it that frequently. But it's all about peace of mind knowing there's only one place I have to go and I can get at it from any computer."

In addition, the system delivers health-related news that is becoming increasing useful to the Schulz family. "My daughter was diagnosed with asthma when she was very young and was aggressively treated for many years," Christy explains. "She grew out of it for a while, but now it's reared its ugly head again."

When Christy first entered some of her daughter's new treatment information into her online file, she noticed that the system was flagging news and recommendations that pertained to her daughter's profile. "The online manager identified some things about my daughter's specific form of treatment and how it might affect her at her exact age," Christy recalls. "I decided to get her involved, showing her how to log on and review the articles that appear. She can read about how her inhaler might make her feel, how to know if it's not working and things to watch for during treatment. It's a great way for her to take an active role in her own health."

Christy was drawn to this particular online approach because it was backed by the Mayo Clinic, a name she trusted. "It makes me think I'm getting good information since it's coming from them. We're often so numb to all of the junk that's put in front of us on the Internet, but this is filtered through this credible channel."

POPULAR ONLINE OPTIONS

There are numerous Web-based record-keeping products currently available, and there are sure to be many more to come in the near future. The underlying goals with most are the same: to offer patients an online storage and data management solution that interacts with physicians and hospitals while linking to the larger online pool of trustworthy health information.

Some services are free; others charge user fees. All promise safety and security on par with online banking systems (although it's never a bad idea to read the fine print to ensure a site's compliance with HIPAA privacy laws).

Microsoft's HealthVault and Google Health are the two main players in this game and with good reason. In my opinion, they are the easiest to use and offer the most valuable features. Brief summaries of both are offered below, along with overviews of two other options. For more details on these products and services, visit their websites. You can also take virtual tours that illustrate how the products are used.

HealthVault (www.HealthVault.com)

HealthVault is Microsoft's contribution to online medical records. This free service has the capacity to store all types of data related to an individual's health and is designed for managing everyday concerns as well as sudden serious diagnoses. Patients (or family members with access to the account) may upload data, images, documents, pharmaceutical records and more. The system also offers electronic connectivity with a growing list of devices (such as blood pressure monitors, treadmills, glucometers) from which it automatically draws data and loads it into the specified account. HealthVault also connects individuals with participating physicians, hospitals, labs and pharmacies.

Sean Nolan, chief architect and general manager of Microsoft's Health Solutions Group, says HealthVault works because it addresses two important challenges: storage and connectivity. "The idea of having consistent and thorough records is obviously important," he says. "But sometimes there are also complicated scenarios such as chronic diseases that have to be managed or adults caring for elderly parents or divorced parents co-managing the health needs of a child. There have been a lot of applications online that tried to offer record-keeping, but they just didn't have uptake. We asked why."

The answer, they found, was that people weren't really connected. Patients could enter data into a Web application but weren't able to integrate it with their care circle (of doctors, family members, nursing centers, pharmacies, etc.). "With HealthVault, people can control the upload of data, they can trust that what's there will stay there and that it will always be accessible," says Nolan. "And we've built the interfaces so the various parties can connect."

In addition, HealthVault provides educational content that relates to a person's health information stored in the system. "Health information is extremely niched," says Nolan. "So we built a system that allows experts to collaborate around this common data store." Patients can receive news and links to online content from doctors and other professionals who deal with their specific health concerns. "People have direct access to the experts in the field who are sharing innovations. That's where you can see the real value in the service," he adds.

Insider's Tip:

Learn the ABCs of medical records. Your personal health record, or PHR, is any official record that relates to your unique medical history. Your personal health information, or PHI, refers to the broader set of information that relates to your health profile.

Google Health (www.google.com/health)

From the search powerhouse comes this free medical record-keeping service for consumers. The goal of Google Health is to simplify the process of maintaining personal health records (PHRs), and to create links between patients and the various members of their health care teams. The service is "untethered" to any one hospital or health care system, so patients can hold on to their electronic medical records even if they change doctors and/or insurance providers. Accounts are password-protected and secure. Patients may fill their Google Health profiles with as much or as little background data as they choose.

Missy Krasner, product marketing manager for Google Health, explains that Google got into the business of PHRs because of the enormous demand for a place to store and organize health information. "We have seen from past surveys in the industry that about one-third of adults have some system of tracking their insurance claims, billing statements, lab tests and other health information," she says. "But only a small percentage of those people are keeping their medical records in a true online format. It will take the health care industry some time to achieve widespread adoption of electronic health records."

So Google stepped in to move things along, building on the successes of the tethered PHR models (such as the very successful online portal offered to Kaiser Permanente patients) to create its untethered model. "We know, statistically, that people change jobs almost every two years, which means that they also change health insurance and sometimes even change doctors," explains Krasner. "Tethered personal health records are great when you're in that system. But the patients don't own that data, and they cannot take it with them if they leave that system because there is no portability of the data."

Google Health, Krasner clarifies, is a patient-centered PHR that offers all the same advantages and more: "It's your data, you control it, you share it when you want to with who you want to."

Dossia (www.dossia.org)

Dossia was founded by a collective of employers and is offered as a free electronic health record service to employees of its participating companies. Individual patients gather their own medical data and upload information to their private accounts to establish a Dossia profile. Physicians and other members of the patients' health care teams can load additional data over time.

PassportMD (www.PassportMD.com)

This fee-based service offers full record-keeping functionality, along with connectivity to physicians and hospitals. It is compatible with Microsoft HealthVault.

Access My Records (www.AccessMy Records.com)

Paying customers of this service receive identification cards that give emergency medical technicians and physicians on-the-spot access to pertinent medical information. The system offers comprehensive online record management and flags the information that health care professionals would need to know in emergency situations. Keychain and wallet cards list the patient's access code, allowing Internet or telephone access to the individual's profile summary.

Insider's Tip:

Create multiple profiles under the umbrella of whatever single system you choose to use. You can manage your own records as well as those of children, elderly parents and friends all in one place.

REAL-WORLD APPLICATIONS

There are countless ways online record-keeping systems can help. Here are a few examples of how patients and family members put them to use:

Back-up copies of tests and images

When a doctor orders a test or image, you want to trust that you'll only have to run it once. By requesting a copy of your test results, radiologist's report or actual films and then posting them to your online records, you drastically reduce the chance of having to re-take the tests because the doctor or hospital loses them. (When you see a new doctor, you will likely be asked to repeat tests for that physician. But storing copies of these "duplicate" results will expand the overall utility of your records.)

Global accessibility

Online records are accessible from any Web-enabled computer or device. So if you're traveling and need medical attention, you (or your proxy) can present useful information to any doctor or hospital with online access.

Medication histories

It's always helpful to have a record of what medications you've taken, what dosages you received and what side effects you may have encountered. Having a comprehensive drug history provides the information to help your present and future doctors avoid negative interactions and dosing errors. There is also growing awareness among cancer survivors of "late effects" – side effects that appear years after cancer-fighting medicines are taken. Having easy access to your medication history could help your doctors help you in the future.

Tracking patterns

Many patients who struggle with food sensitivities and allergies find it helpful to log dietary and reaction patterns. What foods cause stomach upset? During what times of day are gastric issues more prevalent? Which pain relievers are more effective? Tracking such things at home and storing the information in their online records allows patients to offer real data to their doctors, who can then make clinical recommendations.

School forms

When a child's school or summer camp requires a detailed health history, all a parent needs to do is pull up the complete records and print out the pertinent information. No need to look up insurance policy numbers or dates of immunizations or medication dosages. Once these facts and figures are entered, they're always accessible.

Health trends

By recording basic data (weight, body mass index, cholesterol level, resting heart rate, glucose, etc.) and tracking it over time, you can do more than create a complete profile of your health-related stats. You can also watch a visual representation of your own body's trends. For some people, mapping data over time is the best way to stay on track when it comes to health-related targets that they can control through healthy habits.

Remote family access

If a loved one across the country needs medical attention and you are listed as an emergency contact, you can provide health care professionals with life-saving information by summarizing your relative's health history. (This is particularly useful in situations when the person in question is incapacitated.) In addition, you can relay full contact information for your relative's health care team, including the general practitioner and specialists, who might be able to supply crucial supplemental information.

Family histories

Family medical histories are often relevant, so it makes perfect sense to store summaries in your online records. You can include an overview of your relatives' health conditions, specific diseases, age of onset, allergies, drug interactions, etc. as a way of creating a genetic snapshot that might prove useful to you and/or your health care providers.

CUSTOMIZE YOUR SYSTEM

We all have our own ways of doing things based on personal preferences. When managing your health care information, use whatever approach makes you feel in control. For some people, that will mean maintaining everything online; others are more comfortable with hard copies. You can even create a "hybrid" system that combines some of both.

Determine what is most therapeutic for you. Do you prefer plotting graphs by hand or plugging data into a program? Do you want to index the articles you've found on your own or would you rather rely on research conducted by a third party? Do you digest information better when it's on a screen or in a notebook?

The key is to have whatever you need at your fingertips, whether you're reaching for the computer or the bookshelf.

Insider's Tip:

Don't feel pressured to use every single feature of any online records system. Create an à la carte menu that offers what you want.

{ Ten }

Looking Forward to Long-Term Health

Commit to Wellness Once the Crisis Has Passed

In my experience

Those of us who have lived through the nightmare of a serious medical condition have many things in common. We share a keen appreciation for life and health, along with an ever-present worry that illness will one day come knocking on our doors for an unwelcome return visit.

I am certainly no exception. Since I completed my last round of treatment in February 2001, I have felt perfectly healthy and have continued with nothing more than scheduled check-ups with my doctors. I have maintained a normal – some might say slightly fast-paced – professional and personal life. I think of cancer, at this point, as something that I *used* to have.

Still, I do consider it important to check in on the CLL listserv every now and again. The difference is that now, as a survivor, I "lurk" and observe, choosing not to return to my role as a vocal member of the group. When I log on, it is primarily to familiarize myself with the latest buzz about leukemia and to stay on top of the doctors and hospitals generating the patient success stories.

Quite frankly, with my treatment phase behind me, I prefer not to stay as immersed in the "cancer community" as I needed to be during my illness. I want to stay informed, but I want to do so from the perimeter rather than the center of the discussion. I skim the Internet for any CLL-related news and announcements, but I don't devote hours to the search as I once did.

Battling my cancer is no longer part of my daily routine, so there is no clinical need for me to be perfectly up-to-date on the latest developments in CLL research. I also don't think it's good for my emotional makeup to dwell in that place. It took me a few years post-treatment before I could get through a full day without thinking about leukemia. Getting past the stage of feeling like a patient and returning to a normal, healthy life is such a huge part of the process for any of us who have faced a scary diagnosis.

Yes, there's a possibility that my leukemia may return sometime in the future. If that happens, I'll tackle it once again from a position of empowerment. But there's also a possibility that I'll break my leg on a weekend hike up Mt. Rainier. I don't sit and worry about the latter to the point where it stops me from living my life. So why would I obsess about CLL? Right this minute, I am healthy and content. I celebrate every single day.

Insider's Tip:

When it comes to staying informed about your disease category after you've finished treatment, strike a balance between immersion and desertion.

A HEALTHY DOSE OF ONGOING KNOWLEDGE

Congratulations. You've gotten past the hardest part of your journey. Either you've completed treatment and have been declared disease-free or you've successfully entered the management phase of your chronic condition. The most frightening and stressful portion of your ordeal is probably behind you.

Now what?

As an empowered patient, you know how important it is to stay informed. Knowledge served you well when you were in the thick of your illness, and it undoubtedly helped get you to this healthier point. Now you can apply those same skills to your life as a *former* patient.

You can continue to use the strength of the Internet to:

- <u>Stay informed</u>. Remain vigilant in order to stay healthy in the broadest sense.

- <u>Stay empowered</u>. Keep up to date on the latest research related to your condition.

- <u>Stay connected</u>. Know where to go and whom to consult if you have a recurrence.

- <u>Stay helpful</u>. Put your experience to work helping others who are just beginning to face what you did.

- <u>Stay sane</u>. Do what you can to bolster your emotional self and stave off the crazy-making after-effects of illness.

- <u>Stay normal</u>. Return to a wellness regimen to maintain your overall health and prevent common illness.

- <u>Stay celebratory</u>. Congratulate yourself and your support team for a job well done and enjoy every moment of your good health.

Insider's Tip:

When you were ill, you and your doctors made a plan for your treatment. Now it's time to craft a plan for your health.

STAY INFORMED

Ed Greub remembers the moment in late 2005 when his doctor told him the news that would change his life. Ed's doctor had been watching a spot on his left arm for a while and decided to biopsy it when it began to change. With the results in hand, she had Ed come to her office to discuss things. "I went in and she said, 'It's melanoma,'" recalls Ed, who was in his early 70s at the time and busy enjoying his retirement. "And at that point, it was sort of like a blank. I didn't hear anything after that."

When the initial shock wore off, Ed sat down at his computer and did his research. He educated himself on melanoma and checked out the credentials of the oncologist his GP recommended at the nearby university hospital. Within three weeks, he had successful surgery and returned home with his wife.

In the years since, Ed has remained cancer-free, a status he takes very seriously and intends to maintain for a long time to come. Since his diagnosis and surgery, Ed is vigilant about his skin health. "I use a lot of sun block, wear all long-sleeved shirts and wide-brim hats," he reports.

He and his wife even have a monthly ritual they call "P&B" or "pits and boobs." "Once a month, my wife checks her boobs and I check my pits for any swelling in the lymph nodes," says Ed. "My wife pops me on the shoulder at breakfast and says, 'Get in there and check it out.' So I get in there and check it out!"

But Ed's vigilance doesn't end with monthly self-exams. He also commits to staying knowledgeable about his condition and his health. "Once you have something like this, it becomes part of your life," he says. "You can't say it's over. I continue to take care of it, not in a negative way but in a positive, preventive sense."

The Internet, reports Ed, is how he stays informed. "The Web is an integral part of my life. If there's an article I run across on melanoma, I turn to it immediately. I get information from the Melanoma Research Foundation and I pay attention to it."

Being a cancer survivor, in Ed's opinion, is like being a member of Alcoholics Anonymous. "Someone's always going to be an alcoholic whether they're a drinker or a non-drinker," he says. "It's a piece of your life. The last thing you want to do is to bury your head in the sand when it comes to learning what you need to know to stay healthy."

Ed Greub is a living, breathing example of empowerment. The idea is to gather all the wisdom you've gained from your experiences as an empowered patient and put it to use from this point forward to stay as healthy as you can for the rest of your life. Armed with what you've learned, you can enter your post-treatment phase with strength rather than fear.

For some, that will mean turning to the Web for information when your health status changes, even in perfectly innocent ways that have nothing to do with your previous illness (such as when the flu strikes). For others, it will mean managing long-term side effects of medications that are taken to keep illness at bay. (An unfortunate reality of modern medicine is that some life-saving surgical and pharmaceutical interventions introduce new complications that require continued vigilance.)

As the Web grows, the amount of online health-related information will expand. Now that you know how to navigate the millions of pages of available content, you can continue to focus your attention on the sites that can truly assist you. Allow yourself to back off a bit from what was once an intense quest for information, but don't abandon your commitment to knowledge. You might stumble upon something that helps you feel even better than you already do.

Although you are no longer an active patient, doctors and researchers will continue to learn more every day about your disease category, the most effective ways to treat it and the best ways for former patients like you to remain healthy. It's in your best interest to maintain some level of awareness about what they discover.

STAY A SURVIVOR

Increasing attention is being paid to the notion of "survivorship," particularly as it relates to cancer patients. The idea is for doctors and patients alike to manage the post-treatment phase of a person's experience with serious illness and guide

Insider's Tip:

Being a patient, whether you are ill or healthy, is a never-ending condition. The power of information applies in either case.

survivors through the emotional and physical challenges that may emerge down the road.

Visit www.oncolink.org for information about a valuable survivorship program set up by the Institute of Medicine in partnership with the Lance Armstrong Foundation. Called the LiveStrong Care Plan, it helps patients create a summary of their treatments and establish a follow-up care plan that addresses:

- Potential late effects of any treatments received, along with their symptoms and recommended treatments
- Recommendations for future cancer screening for recurrence or new primary sites
- Psychosocial effects of cancer and survivorship, including relationships and sexuality/fertility
- Financial issues

- Recommendations for a healthy lifestyle
- Genetic counseling (if applicable)
- Effective prevention options
- Referrals for follow-up care
- Support resources

Insider's Tip:

It is much easier to review news and information about your health concern when you're not motivated by fear.

STAY EMPOWERED

Back when you were new to patienthood, you most likely tiptoed into your research to avoid feeling overwhelmed by the enormity of it all. Now that you're an experienced and powerful patient, you are better equipped to take a more aggressive approach. Your job right now is to stay healthy. You can do that by digesting more sophisticated online content.

Empowered patients can employ some of these approaches to take control of the rest of their healthy lives:

- **<u>Review research papers</u>**. You are now quite familiar with the common terms used to describe and discuss your health condition. The research is ongoing. Why not stay informed by reading clinical papers? Even a quick review of an article's abstract (summary statement) will reveal the latest findings. You might even learn something that applies to your current post-treatment phase.

- **<u>Look at medical conference agendas</u>**. By now you probably know the names and websites of professional medical associations that educate physicians specializing in your health concern. You may have already reviewed some of their online content. Why stop now? Stay on top of what these specialists consider the most important topics in their field by clicking through to their upcoming meeting links and reviewing the agendas. Whatever they plan to discuss at their next professional gathering is the hot topic in that area of medicine.

- **<u>Attend medical conferences</u>**. You might attend a local or national meeting of physicians who will gather to discuss your disease category. These events are typically open to anyone who has an interest in the topic (not restricted to doctors only). You'll hear about the latest research findings at the same time as the medical specialists. You'll also have a prime networking opportunity that could pay real dividends in the future.

- **<u>Ask to speak at a medical conference</u>**. An increasing number of patients are speaking to audiences of medical professionals to convey the other side of the health care experience. If you feel you have an important story to tell, discuss with your physician the possibility of speaking at a conference or contact a medical association directly.

Insider's Tip:

Don't dwell on "what ifs." Stay focused on "what is."

STAY CONNECTED

Sometimes former patients who are years past treatment have to deal with the cruel reality of recurrence. It can happen to anybody, even the most empowered.

That was the experience of Michael Kurzawski, a former Marine and Vietnam veteran from the Midwest. Throughout his adult life, Michael had dealt with various health issues, including rheumatoid arthritis. Then, in the late 1990s, he was diagnosed with cancer in his cheek. Michael's doctors recommended a course of treatment that included radiation therapy. Following his treatment, Michael was declared cancer-free.

Nearly ten years later, in January 2009, Michael received devastating news. Not only was his cancer back, but it was back with a vengeance. Doctors reported that he had stage IV cancer in his cheek (the original site), as well as in his jawbone.

"The diagnosis wasn't too good because of my other health issues, like my rheumatoid arthritis," he says. "I couldn't open my mouth very wide. The oncologist didn't give me much of a shot at surgery."

Michael was given four months to live and sent on his way.

But he and his family were not willing to accept such a dire prognosis. They got to work researching his options, going online to learn more about his condition. Their goal was to find out which doctors and hospitals were address-ing cancers such as Michael's and where patients with recur-rence had a better chance of survival.

Based on what he and his family learned, Michael ended up at a leading Midwest hospital, whose doctors identified him as a candidate for surgery – not just to remove the can-cer but also to reconstruct his diseased jaw.

When I interviewed Michael for a Patient Power pro-gram, he had already recovered from his successful surgery. Better yet, he had exceeded what his first oncologist had predicted would be his life expectancy. To Michael, it was a simple matter of looking to see what other doctors knew about his condition and pursuing their expertise.

When asked what he would say to others in a similar situation, Michael declares, "You've got to give it your best shot and you just have to try to prolong your life. That's the main thing. I did it for my family and myself."

Michael's story is a cautionary tale with a happy ending. If your disease recurs, the chances are pretty good that medical science has improved since the last time you faced this condition. The Web can help you conduct preliminary research so you can get yourself up to date on the latest news and discoveries related to your diagnosis. It's also possible that you'll need to turn to a new doctor or health care team when returning to patienthood. Be open and flexible now, just as you were the first time around.

Insider's Tip:

If you're diagnosed with a recurrence, remember that research has continued while your disease was away, likely resulting in new approaches and treatments.

Stay helpful

Like most new moms, Brenda Winiarski was overjoyed by the arrival of her daughter, Molly, in 2000. "She looked just like the Gerber baby – chubby and the picture of health," Brenda recalls. "We were walking on air."

But just six days into their life as a family, Brenda and her husband received an urgent call. Molly's newborn screening test results had come back and there was a problem. Molly had tested positive for phenylketonuria (PKU), a rare genetic metabolic disorder. The Winiarskis were told that if their daughter did not follow a medically restricted low-protein diet for the rest of her life, she could sustain serious neurological damage.

Brenda studied up on PKU and quickly learned that Molly and other PKU sufferers are unable to break down a specific amino acid found in protein called phenylalanine ("phe"). She researched how to measure and calculate the amount of phe Molly's system could handle daily. Brenda found plenty of resources on what ingredients to include and restrict in her daughter's diet, but she found very little about what meals to serve. The greatest challenge, she figured out, would be cooking dishes that Molly would want to eat.

"I looked into my baby's eyes and promised her that PKU was not going to get in the way of her enjoyment of food," Brenda says. "I soon realized that this promise meant that I had to take on a job I never expected (and, honestly, one for which I was not qualified): personal chef."

So after five years of coping with the challenges of PKU, Brenda went off to culinary school when Molly went off to kindergarten. She was determined to learn how to create family meals that would be as delicious as they were healthy. Then she did even more. Along with another mom whose child has PKU, Brenda created a website called Cook for Love (www.cookforlove.org). This non-profit enterprise seeks to empower families dealing with PKU; it offers recipes, support and resources to help manage the challenges posed by the condition.

Her determination and resourcefulness prompted Brenda to accomplish more than her primary goal of supporting Molly. Her work, and that of her Cook for Love team, has enabled families all over the world to tackle the daily grind of living with PKU. Better yet, the site helps what she calls an "underserved population" experience the joy of food.

Brenda is impressed by how PKU doesn't define her daughter. "When you look at Molly, you can't help but admire her," says her proud mom. "She's one of those kids who's so determined and so powerful."

Brenda's story is a great example of how to turn a health crisis into a philanthropic mission. Rather than dwell in anger about having to parent a child with a serious medical condition, Brenda found a way not just to manage her own family's needs but to assist countless other families at the same time.

Anyone can take a similar approach. Whatever the health concern, you can use what you have learned to help others who may just be starting out on their journey. You've walked in their shoes and you offer a powerful perspective. Some survivors even consider this to be nothing less than their responsibility.

I field calls and emails daily from terrified patients and family members, and I can attest to the exhilaration of guiding people toward potentially life-saving information.

Consider a few ideas of how to share your hard-won wealth of knowledge via the Web:

- Become a member or owner of a listserv devoted to your disease category.
- Volunteer as a "knowledge provider" in online communities.
- Consider patient advocacy.
- Blog or Twitter about your experiences as a former patient and a survivor.
- Post video testimonies to tell your story.
- Participate in online talk shows.
- Seek out clinical trials that follow survivors.

Insider's Tip:

Turn your negative experience into a positive by spreading the power of information to others.

Stay sane

It is perfectly normal to want to move past your illness. You devoted an enormous amount of time and energy to your case while you were in the middle of it. Now you might just want to leave it – and all of its online buzz – behind you. This is your prerogative.

But if you take this approach, make sure not to bury your head in the sand to avoid any mention of your former disease. Blissful ignorance is one thing. But if you find your-self working hard to steer clear of the mere mention of your condition, staying informed might make you feel more in control. The trick is to be stronger than the illness.

Insider's Tip:

You'll drive yourself nuts if you assume every abnormality is a sign of recurrence or of some new serious problem. Address headaches, fatigue and other everyday symptoms as annoyances unless they become out of hand.

STAY NORMAL

Patients who have successfully battled a life-threatening illness sometimes begin to feel immune to the rest of life's little medical nuisances. Sadly, nobody is. Even those of us who proudly wave the survivor flag must remember to pay attention to the rest of our bodies.

Now that you know how to use the Web to tackle life-threatening conditions, return to it to manage the everyday stuff. You may find it surprisingly refreshing to search for information related to weight management, heart health or flu shots. You've returned to the general population of healthy people, so you've earned the privilege (some might call it a burden) of taking care of your whole health.

Type 1 diabetes patients still need colonoscopies. Women who have gotten their rheumatoid arthritis under control still need mammograms. Leukemia survivors must still watch for signs of high cholesterol. Celebrate the normalcy of your status by protecting your overall good health.

Turn to the Web to find helpful tips on general and preventive health. I think MayoClinic.com and EverydayHealth.com are the best such sites, but there are numerous others that provide similar information.

Insider's Tip:

Put your Web wisdom to work for preventive purposes.

STAY CELEBRATORY

The one silver lining to medical crisis is that it helps us remember how precious life and good health are. Celebrate your healthy status by "seizing the day." It's highly beneficial.

If you've been declared disease-free, acknowledge this important milestone. Throw a party, plant a tree or have a ceremonial burial of your hospital ID bracelet. If your condition is chronic, treat yourself to frequent subtle reminders of the work you've done to get yourself to this place. Pat yourself on the back for keeping your medication log so well organized; take note of how well you can explain the science of your condition to the uninitiated. In short, do whatever it takes to reward yourself and those who love you for all the work devoted to getting you back to health.

Enjoy each and every day that takes you farther away from uncontrolled illness and involve your family and friends in the celebration. I sure do.

Afterword

Perspectives on Mortality

Most people's childhood memories of illness center on being sick, receiving medicine and getting well. I remember Dr. Landis, our family doctor, sitting on the edge of my bed (back in the day when doctors made house calls) and reaching into his black doctor's bag, pulling out a small bottle of cherry-flavored cough syrup and giving it to me to drink. I soon felt better.

If only getting well were always so simple! If only treatments were so available and foolproof!

Reality sets in as we age. There are children and adults who get seriously ill – and some "don't make it." There are friends and relatives who get sick and never recover. Some die suddenly, while others succumb after periods of long illness.

As you read this, you are propelled toward something somewhere on the Internet that might offer up a better answer for yourself or a loved one. Maybe there's a smarter doctor, a brand new treatment, a promising clinical trial, a patient who has a secret that can make all the difference. Yes, in the millions of pages on the Web, there is that chance.

But then you may need to step back and accept the possibility that all that can be done has been done. We are mortal. Life is a "terminal condition." There may not be an answer that's any better than what you've already been told. Mortality becomes a looming reality.

Here's a story from my own family. It's about a relative in her 60s who became sick while on a cruise. The diagnosis that came back eventually could not have been worse: pancreatic cancer. Yona Kollin, a therapist, wife of a prominent rabbi, mother and grandmother had wide support to "get the best." And she did. She was fortunate to be a candidate for a state-of-the-art surgical procedure that would cut out the cancer and give her a chance at survival. While complications from the surgery almost killed her, Yona went back to a fairly normal life for five-and-a-half years.

I write this just a few weeks after we learned that the cancer had returned – with a vengeance. The whole family accompanied Yona and her husband to a major cancer research center. The pancreatic cancer specialist there told her there was nothing to do except help her be comfortable as death approached within a month or two. Terrible news.

"What about clinical trials?" her daughter asked. Yes, they were told. There may be a trial in the Philippines (the family was in Los Angeles). But would Yona be well enough to travel? Would she be a good candidate for the trial? Would it work? Was it wasting precious time with family and diminishing her quality of life?

Yona opted not to go and urged her daughter to stop combing the Internet for any glimmer of an option. Instead, she wanted to make videos for her children and grandchildren. And she wanted the one child with an upcoming bat mitzvah (at age 13), still months away, to deliver a preview performance early for Grandma. These shared gifts and experiences would be blessings for all.

Unfortunately, Yona died 10 days before her granddaughter's bat mitzvah. She died in her own bed with close family by her side. Her dying wish was that the upcoming family celebration proceed. And it did. We all felt her presence with us and young Kayla surely made Grandma very proud.

There is a time to stop the quest for new information and accept mortality. As far as medical science has come, there is still so far for it to go. Illness will take lives away from all of us. Our own lives too will end some day.

So while I am a tremendous believer that "knowledge is power" and familiar with the many ways the Internet can help make us smarter and healthier, it can only do so much even when it is used wisely.

We must try hard to use this powerful digital-age tool to its utmost. Then there comes a time when we must surrender and face the end with dignity and grace.

A Note About Our Powerful Patients

Each of the patients profiled or mentioned in this book has been featured on a Patient Power program or been interviewed by one of the book's authors. Their stories are real, although some names have been changed at the patients' request. Please feel free to review full interviews in audio, video or text format at www.patientpower.info.

We are enormously indebted to the following patients, caregivers, friends and dedicated professionals: Beth Mays, Charlie Mays, Charlie Jennings, Jill Peterson, Lynne Matallana, Matthew Zachary, Mike McKelheer, Patricia Beck, Rob Beck, Ed Edwards, Gretchen Cover, Karen Reynolds, Cooper Reynolds, David Nudelman, David Serkin-Poole, Barb Lackritz, Jennifer Ambrose, Barry Anderson, Dave deBronkart, Cathi Little, Amy Gray, Rachel Daniels, Lindsay Wolfe, Katie Bunker, Patricia Dunlap, Eitan Schorr, Ruth Schorr, Esther Schorr,

Valerie Fraser, Josh Freedman, Dr. Elizabeth Morrison, Dr. Sarah Simpson, Sara McKenzie, Christy Schulz, Sean Nolan, Missy Krasner, Ed Greub, Michael Kurzawski, Brenda Winiarski, Molly Winiarski.

Health-Related Websites and Other Online Resources

Throughout this book, we have listed the online addresses of numerous websites that patients might find useful in their quest for information and power. Most of these resources, and many others, are explored further in the online pages of Patient Power at www.PatientPower.info.

We invite you to visit Patient Power and browse its programs and get to know some of its powerful patients. We encourage you to join the discussion if you're comfortable doing so. Whatever disease category you identify with, you'll find stories and points of view that will remind you of your own. There is a large community of like-minded patients awaiting your arrival.

INDEX

Acknowledgements

This book has been in the works for several years, and the road to publishing it has been a winding one. Along the way, the focused team that has supported the project has helped keep it on track toward the goal of publication. There are plenty of thanks to go around.

Amy Gray's inspiration planted the seeds for the project, and the book would not have come to be without her initial vision. Blake Shewey, Patient Power producer extraordinaire, was in the trenches with us as we planned, wrote, revised and completed the book, and her contributions are evident on every page. John Marshall offered valuable editorial suggestions, and our words read more clearly because of his efforts. Alice Acheson gave us her publishing expertise, which helped define our strategies. Barbara Lowenstein believed in this book and encouraged its publication, even in the face of significant industry change. Brian Blankinship contributed his technical and artistic support in the final stretch. Thanks too to the CreateSpace team for guiding us through the process and expressing enthusiasm for what's written here.

We are also grateful to the patients, family members and medical personnel who have contributed their ideas and stories. They are true heroes in the fight for better health and health care in the Internet age.

Lastly, this book could not have taken shape without the support of our spouses, Esther Schorr and Kevin Thomas. They are just as committed to helping you benefit from this Insider's Guide as we are. They have our love for their devotion to us and to you.

Your purchase of *The Web-Savvy Patient* is testimony to the fact that there was an audience waiting for what we had to say. This book is an offering of the new non-profit health communications organization, the Patient Empowerment Network (PEN), founded by Andrew and Esther Schorr. Its goal is to give American consumers the tools to be in control of their health and health care, whether or not they are active patients. The PEN also aims to accredit health care organizations as to whether they meet a standard of honoring, respecting and encouraging their patients to be empowered. By purchasing this book, you are helping the PEN take flight.

We hope you find value in *The Web-Savvy Patient,* and we welcome your comments and stories of how it made a difference for you or a loved one. Write to us any time at comments@WebSavvyPatient.com.

Andrew Schorr
Mary Adam Thomas

Author Profiles

Andrew Schorr is a pioneer in Internet health and medical programs who became a patient himself, participating in a clinical trial and surviving leukemia. This followed 25 years as a reporter, producer and national reality television programmer. Andrew began his broadcasting career at WBTV in Charlotte, N.C., and then became a national producer of Westinghouse Broadcasting's PM/Evening Magazine, the nation's number one syndicated television show and one of the first reality programs. Based in Los Angeles and later in Seattle, he produced award-winning national cable television medical documentaries and patient education videos. Along with his wife, Esther, Andrew helped produce a daily national television program, Group One Medical. He produced over 100 health and medical education videos. Andrew also invented telephone talk shows for patients and later was among the first to produce live webcasts for patients. He has been honored by many groups for his innovation in health communications and his devotion to helping other patients.

He is the founder of Patient Power, an online patient education resource located at www.PatientPower.info and the co-founder of the Patient Empowerment Network located at www.PowerfulPatients.org. He lives in Mercer Island, Washington.

Mary Adam Thomas is a freelance writer who has been involved in health care communications since the 1980s. Her broad portfolio of written work, which has appeared in print and online, includes patient education resources, promotional material and editorial articles for both clinical and consumer audiences. Her professional experience extends into the fields of green design and development, parenting, elder care, banking and finance, real estate, interior design and recreational product manufacturing. Mary is also the collaborative author, with Jason F. McLennan, of *Zugunruhe:The Inner Migration to Profound Environmental Change* (Ecotone Publishing). She lives in the Seattle area with her husband and two children.